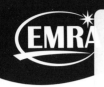

PressorDex

2nd Edition

John C. Greenwood, MD
Editor-In-Chief
University of Maryland
Department of Medicine, Division of Pulmonary & Critical Care

Disclaimer

This handbook is intended as a general guide to therapy only. While the editors have taken reasonable measures to ensure the accuracy of drug and dosing information used in this guide, the user is encouraged to consult other resources or consultants when necessary to confirm appropriate therapy, side effects, interactions, and contraindications. The publisher, authors, editors, and sponsoring organizations specifically disclaim any liability for any omissions or errors found in this handbook, for appropriate use, or treatment errors. Furthermore, although this handbook is as comprehensive as possible, the vast differences in emergency practice settings may necessitate treatment approaches other than presented here.

Copyright ©2015
Emergency Medicine Residents' Association
1125 Executive Circle, Irving, TX 75038-2522
972.550.0920
www.emra.org

ISBN 978-1-929854-36-3

2014-2015 EMRA Board of Directors

Editors

Editor-In-Chief
John C. Greenwood, MD
Fellow, Division of Pulmonary & Critical Care Medicine
University of Maryland School of Medicine
Baltimore, MD
Email: johncgreenwood@gmail.com

Senior Editors
Lillian L. Emlet, MD, MS, FACEP
Assistant Professor
Program Director, EM-CCM Fellowship of the MCCTP
Departments of Critical Care Medicine & Emergency Medicine
University of Pittsburgh School of Medicine
Pittsburgh, PA

Haney A. Mallemat, MD
Assistant Professor of Emergency Medicine
University of Maryland School of Medicine
Baltimore, MD

Michael E. Winters, MD, FACEP, FAAEM
Associate Professor of Emergency Medicine & Medicine
Co-Director, Combined EM/IM/Critical Care Program
University of Maryland School of Medicine
Baltimore, MD

Associate Editor
Michael T. McCurdy, MD
Assistant Professor of Pulmonary, Critical Care Medicine & Emergency Medicine
Program Director, Critical Care Medicine Fellowship
University of Maryland School of Medicine
Baltimore, MD

EMRA Staff Editor
Rachel Donihoo
Emergency Medicine Residents' Assocation

Contributing Editors

Timothy J. Ellender, MD
Assistant Professor
Co-Director, Critical Care Fellowship
Department of Emergency Medicine
Indiana University School of Medicine
Indianapolis, IN

Bryan D. Hayes, PharmD, DABAT
Clinical Specialist, Emergency Medicine & Toxicology
Manager, Emergency Medicine Pharmacy Services
University of Maryland Medical Center
Clinical Assistant Professor
University of Maryland School of Medicine/School of Pharmacy
Baltimore, MD

Le N. Lu, MD, MS
Clinical Assistant Professor of Emergency Medicine
Director, Pediatric Emergency Medicine Education
Department of Emergency Medicine
University of Maryland School of Medicine
Baltimore, MD

Evie Marcolini, MD, FACEP, FAAEM
Assistant Professor
Departments of Emergency Medicine & Neurology
Divisions of Neurocritical Care & Emergency Neurology & Surgical Critical Care
Yale University School of Medicine
New Haven, CT

Anand Swaminathan, MD, MPH, FACEP, FAAEM
Assistant Professor of Emergency Medicine
Assistant Residency Director, Emergency Medicine
NYU/Bellevue
New York, NY

Foreword

It is a pleasure to present the second edition of the *PressorDex*. First and foremost, it is important to thank everyone for their tireless efforts in writing, editing, and creating this manual. Without these contributors, this project would never have been possible.

It's amazing how in just two short years so much has changed. This edition has incorporated therapeutic options based on a number of new and exciting studies regarding pulmonary embolism, anticoagulation, anticoagulation reversal, as well as many others. The *PressorDex* was inspired by our sickest patients – those we take care of every day in both our emergency departments and intensive care units. Our goal was to create a therapeutic guide to the myriad of pressors, vasoactive agents, and continuous infusions these patients require. Choosing the appropriate medications and dosing regimens can often become complicated – especially during a busy shift. We hope that this book will improve the care of those critically ill patients and also help educate those who use it.

The *PressorDex* continues to be a multidisciplinary collaboration of emergency medicine-trained residents, critical care fellows, attending physicians, and clinical pharmacologists across the United States. Each of the following chapters has been written by an emergency medicine-trained physician. The editorial staff was unanimously impressed by the quality of each chapter, which reinforced our belief that emergency medicine physicians do an amazing job of taking care of critically ill patients.

Appropriate and Responsible Use: The *PressorDex* is designed to be a quick, easy-to-use reference and should not be used for diagnosis or as a comprehensive treatment manual for any specific disease process. This guide is not intended to be a definitive reference text. When initiating any of the recommended medications, it is important to consider all of its possible relative and absolute contraindications.

The medications listed in this handbook are highly dependent on the editors' choices and may differ based on practice location. Some individual indications for other medications might have been omitted from this text. In cases with multiple pharmacologic options, we have chosen medications with the most data on efficacy or that are the least expensive. If the medication choices were all considered equivalent, they were simply listed in alphabetical order. We have made every attempt to use specialty-specific guidelines and peer-reviewed publications for each indication.

It is our goal that every medication and dosage is as accurate as possible, and we have made every attempt to avoid typographical errors. Individual patient conditions should be taken into account with each medication that is administered. Alterations in dosing may be required for patients with renal or hepatic dysfunction.

Contributors

All contributors are emergency medicine-trained residents or fellows.

SEDATION

Jonathan S. Auerbach, MD
Fellow, Department of Critical Care
Medicine
University of Pittsburgh Medical Center
Pittsburgh, PA

Katelin Engerer, MD
Resident Physician
Department of Emergency Medicine
Dartmouth Hitchcock Medical Center
Lebanon, NH

PARALYTICS

Jonathan Elmer, MD
Assistant Professor
Departments of Critical Care Medicine
& Emergency Medicine
University of Pittsburgh Medical Center
Pittsburgh, PA

David Yamane, MD
Resident Physician
Department of Emergency Medicine
Massachusetts General Hospital &
Brigham and Woman's Hospital
Boston, MA

CARDIOVASCULAR

Abdominal Aortic Aneurysm

Brandon Quarles, MD
Resident Physician
Department of Emergency Medicine
New York University/Bellevue
Hospital Center
New York, NY

Annalee Baker, MD
Attending Physician
Department of Emergency Medicine
New York University School of Medicine
New York, NY

Acute Coronary Syndrome

Semhar Tewelde, MD
Assistant Professor
Department of Emergency Medicine
University of Maryland School of
Medicine
Baltimore, MD

Aortic Dissection

Bethany Radin, DO
Fellow, Division of Pulmonary &
Critical Care Medicine
University of Maryland Medical Center
Baltimore, MD

Michael Allison, MD
Chair, EMRA Critical Care Division
Fellow, Division of Pulmonary &
Critical Care Medicine
University of Maryland Medical Center
Baltimore, MD

Atrial Fibrillation with RVR

Connor Lundy, MD
Attending Physician
The Permanente Medical Group
San Francisco, CA

Congestive Heart Failure

John C. Greenwood, MD
Fellow, Division of Pulmonary &
Critical Care Medicine
University of Maryland Medical Center
Baltimore, MD

Hypertensive Emergency

Ari Kestler, MD
Attending Physician
Department of Emergency Medicine
Regional Medical Center of San Jose
San Jose, CA

Supraventricular Tachycardia

Jennifer Chang, MD
Attending Physician
Department of Emergency Medicine
University of Maryland
    Upper Chesapeake Hospital
Baltimore, MD

Nick Santavicca, MD
Resident Physician
Departments of Emergency Medicine &
    Internal Medicine
University of Maryland Medical Center
Baltimore, MD

Ventricular Tachycardia

Emily Gundert, MD
Fellow, Department of Emergency
    Medicine & Division of
    Pulmonary Critical Care Medicine
Indiana University School of Medicine
Indianapolis, IN

CENTRAL NERVOUS SYSTEM
Acute Ischemic Stroke

Josh Keegan, MD
Resident Physician
Department of Emergency Medicine
Yale University School of Medicine
New Haven, CT

Wan-Tsu W. Chang, MD
Assistant Professor
Department of Emergency Medicine
University of Maryland School of
    Medicine
Baltimore, MD

Aneurysmal Subarachnoid Hemorrhage

Natalie Kreitzer, MD
Fellow, Division of Neurocritical Care
University of Cincinnati Medical Center
Cincinnati, OH

Wan-Tsu W. Chang, MD
Assistant Professor
Department of Emergency Medicine
University of Maryland School of Medicine
Baltimore, MD

Cerebral Edema

Vi Am Dinh, MD
Assistant Professor
Departments of Emergency Medicine &
    Internal Medicine
Division of Critical Care
Loma Linda University Medical Center
Loma Linda, CA

Michelle Iwaki, MD
Chief Resident
Department of Emergency Medicine
Loma Linda University Medical Center
Loma Linda, CA

Status Epilepticus

Katrina Harper-Kirksey, MD
Fellow, Division of Anesthesia
    Critical Care Medicine
Stanford Hospital and Clinics
Stanford, CA

Eric Steinberg, MD
Attending Physician
Department of Emergency Medicine
Staten Island University Hospital
Staten Island, NY

Traumatic Spinal Cord Injury

Cindy H. Hsu, MD, PhD
Fellow, Trauma/Surgical Critical Care
R. Adams Cowley Shock Trauma Center
University of Maryland Medical Center
Baltimore, MD

ENDOCRINE-METABOLIC
Diabetic Ketoacidosis

Colleen Stoeppel, MD
Assistant Professor
Department of Surgery
Division of Trauma/Critical Care
UT Southwestern – Parkland Memorial
    Hospital
Dallas, TX

Christopher Couch, MD
Fellow, Surgical Critical Care
Methodist Health System
Dallas, TX

Hypernatremia
Benjamin Cleary, MD
Resident Physician
Department of Emergency Medicine
New York University/Bellevue
   Hospital Center
New York, NY

Hyponatremia
Keegan Tupchong, MD
Chief Resident
Department of Emergency Medicine
New York University/Bellevue
   Hospital Center
New York, NY

Anand Swaminathan, MD
Assistant Professor/Assistant Residency
   Director
Department of Emergency Medicine
New York University/Bellevue
   Hospital Center
New York, NY

Neuroleptic Malignant Syndrome
William Scheels, MD
Resident Physician
Department of Emergency Medicine
University of Pittsburgh Medical Center
Pittsburgh, PA

GASTROINTESTINAL
Mesenteric Ischemia
Amy Panzenbeck, MD
Resident Physician
Department of Emergency Medicine
New York University/Bellevue
   Hospital Center
New York, NY

Jeff Pepin, MD
Assistant Professor
Department of Emergency Medicine
University of Minnesota
Minneapolis, MN

Upper GI Bleed
David Hackenson, MD
Fellow, Department of Emergency
   Medicine
Division of Pulmonary/Critical Care
   Medicine
Indiana University School of Medicine
Indianapolis, IN

Timothy Ellender, MD
Assistant Professor
Co-Director, Critical Care Fellowship
Department of Emergency Medicine
Indiana University School of Medicine
Indianapolis, IN

HEMATOLOGY-ONCOLOGY
Anticoagulation
Mark J. Conroy, MD
Fellow, Department of Emergency
   Medicine
University of Pittsburgh Medical Center
Pittsburgh, PA

Jacqueline Roth, MD
Resident Physician
Department of Emergency Medicine
University of Pittsburgh Medical Center
Pittsburgh, PA

Anticoagulation Reversal
Jeremiah Escajeda, MD
Fellow, Department of Emergency
   Medicine
University of Pittsburgh Medical Center
Pittsburgh, PA

James Boulden, MD
Resident Physician
Department of Emergency Medicine
University of Pittsburgh Medical Center
Pittsburgh, PA

Coagulopathy Reversal
Michael Buscher, DO
Fellow, Department of Critical Care
   Medicine
University of Pittsburgh Medical Center
Pittsburgh, PA

Tumor Lysis Syndrome
Phil Magidson, MD, MPH
Resident Physician
Departments of Emergency Medicine &
Internal Medicine
University of Maryland Medical Center
Baltimore, MD

Adam Brenner, MD
Fellow, Departments of Emergency
Medicine & Internal Medicine
University of Maryland Medical Center
Baltimore, MD

IMMUNOLOGY
Anaphylaxis
Sarah Dubbs, MD
Clinical Instructor
Department of Emergency Medicine
University of Maryland School of
Medicine
Baltimore, MD

Megan Cobb, MD
Resident Physician
Departments of Emergency Medicine &
Pediatrics
University of Maryland Medical Center
Baltimore, MD

OBSTETRICS & GYNECOLOGY
Eclampsia
Zach Dezman, MD, MS
Clinical Research Fellow
Department of Emergency Medicine
University of Maryland School of
Medicine
Baltimore, MD

Michael Scott, MD
Fellow, Pulmonary & Critical Care
Medicine
University of Maryland Medical Center
Baltimore, MD

PULMONARY
Pulmonary Arterial Hypertension
Diego Casali, MD
Fellow, Division of Pulmonary & Critical
Care Medicine
Washington University School
of Medicine
St. Louis, MO

Evan Leibner, MD
Resident Physician
Department of Emergency Medicine
Stony Brook University Medical Center
Stony Brook, NY

Pulmonary Embolism
Nick Johnson, MD
Fellow, Division of Pulmonary & Critical
Care Medicine
University of Washington
Seattle, WA

Kevin Scott, MD
Assistant Professor
Department of Emergency Medicine
University of Pennsylvania
Philadelphia, PA

Status Asthmaticus
Krystle Shafer, MD
Resident Physician
Department of Emergency Medicine
Wellspan York Hospital
York, PA

Meagan Cooper, DO
Resident Physician
Department of Emergency Medicine
Wellspan York Hospital
York, PA

Sepsis
Michael Scott, MD
Fellow, Pulmonary & Critical Care
Medicine
University of Maryland Medical Center
Baltimore, MD

Zach Dezman, MD, MS
Clinical Research Fellow
Department of Emergency Medicine
University of Maryland School of Medicine
Baltimore, MD

TOXICOLOGY

Acetaminophen Overdose

Rachel Wightman, MD
Resident Physician
Department of Emergency Medicine
New York University School of Medicine
New York, NY

Anand Swaminathan, MD, MPH
Assistant Professor/Assistant Residency
    Director
Department of Emergency Medicine
New York University/Bellevue
    Hospital Center
New York, NY

Alcohol Withdrawal

Maite Huis in 't Veld, MD
Resident Physician
Department of Emergency Medicine
University of Maryland Medical Center
Baltimore, MD

Elizabeth Kenez, MD
Fellow, Emergency Ultrasound
Department of Emergency Medicine
MedStar Washington Hospital Center/
    Georgetown University Hospital
Washington, DC

Anticholinergic Toxicity

Jessica Hetherington Lopez, MD
Resident Physician
Department of Emergency Medicine
New York University School of Medicine
New York, NY

David Jang, MD, MSC
K12 Scholar, National Heart, Lung
    & Blood Institute
Department of Emergency Medicine
University of Pennsylvania
Perelman School of Medicine
Philadelphia, PA

Beta-Blocker Overdose

Gregg Chesney, MD
Assistant Professor
Division of Adult Critical Care Services &
    Department of Emergency Medicine
Maimonides Medical Center/Albert
    Einstein College of Medicine
Brooklyn, NY

Akhila Pamula, MD
Resident Physician
Department of Emergency Medicine
Stanford Hospital and Clinics
Stanford, CA

Calcium-Channel Blocker Overdose

Adaira Landry, MD
Resident Physician
Department of Emergency Medicine
New York University School of Medicine
New York, NY

Anand Swaminathan, MD, MPH
Assistant Professor/Assistant Residency
    Director
Department of Emergency Medicine
New York University/Bellevue
    Hospital Center
New York, NY

Cholinergic Crisis

Xiao Chi (Tony) Zhang, MD
Resident Physician
Department of Emergency Medicine
Alpert Medical School – Brown
    University
Providence, RI

Chad Van Ginkel, MD
Resident Physician
Department of Emergency Medicine
Alpert Medical School – Brown
    University
Providence, RI

Cyanide Toxicity
Jose V. Nable, MD, MS, NRP
Attending Physician
Department of Emergency Medicine
MedStar Georgetown University Hospital
Georgetown University School of Medicine
Washington, DC

Elizabeth Kenez, MD
Fellow, Emergency Ultrasound
Department of Emergency Medicine
MedStar Washington Hospital Center/
  Georgetown University Hospital
Washington, DC

Digoxin Toxicity
Michael Allison, MD
Chair, EMRA Critical Care Division
Fellow, Pulmonary & Critical Care Medicine
University of Maryland School of Medicine
Baltimore, MD

Bethany Radin, DO
Fellow, Division of Pulmonary &
  Critical Care Medicine
University of Maryland Medical Center
Baltimore, MD

Hydrofluoric Acid Toxicity
Eric Steinberg, MD
Attending Physician
Department of Emergency Medicine
Staten Island University Hospital
Staten Island, NY

Matthew Colantoni, MD
Resident Physician
Department of Emergency Medicine
Mount Sinai Beth Israel
New York, NY

Opioid Overdose
Fereshteh Sani, MD
Resident Physician
Department of Emergency Medicine
New York University/Bellevue
  Hospital Center
New York, NY

Christopher Caspers, MD
Assistant Professor
Department of Emergency Medicine
New York University/Bellevue
  Hospital Center
New York, NY

Oral Hypoglycemic Overdose
Donald E. Stader III, MD
Attending Physician
Department of Emergency Medicine
Salem Emergency Physician
  Services, PC
Salem, OR

James Dazhe Cao, MD
Fellow, Medical Toxicology
Department of Emergency Medicine
Denver Health and Hospital
Denver, CO

Pit-Viper Envenomation
Katherine Baugher, DO
Attending Physician
Department of Emergency Medicine
MedStar Franklin Square Hospital
  Center
Baltimore, MD

Tu Carol Nguyen, DO
Resident Physician
Department of Emergency Medicine
University of Maryland Medical Center
Baltimore, MD

Salicylate Overdose
Danya Khoujah, MBBS
Assistant Professor
Department of Emergency Medicine
University of Maryland School of
  Medicine
Baltimore, MD

Tareq Al-Salamah, MBBS
Resident Physician
Department of Emergency Medicine
University of Maryland Medical Center
Baltimore, MD

Toxic Alcohol Ingestion
Christopher K. Schott, MD, MS
Assistant Professor
Departments of Emergency Medicine
   & Critical Care Medicine
University of Pittsburgh Medical Center
Pittsburgh, PA

Jeremiah Escajeda, MD
Fellow, Department of Emergency
   Medicine
University of Pittsburgh Medical Center
Pittsburgh, PA

Tricyclic Antidepressant Overdose
Michael Buscher, DO
Fellow, Department of Critical Care
   Medicine
University of Pittsburgh Medical Center
Pittsburgh, PA

PEDIATRICS
Cardiogenic Shock
Joey M. Scollan, DO
Attending Physician
Departments of Emergency Medicine
   & Pediatrics
Elliot Hospital
Manchester, NH

Danielle Devereaux, MD
Attending Physician
Departments of Emergency Medicine
   & Pediatrics
Prince George Hospital Center
Cheverly, MD

Septic Shock
Ashley Strobel, MD
Chief Resident
Emergency Medicine & Pediatrics
   Combined Residency
University of Maryland Medical Center
Baltimore, MD

Michael Holdsworth, MD
Resident Physician
Emergency Medicine & Pediatrics
   Combined Residency
University of Maryland Medical Center
Baltimore, MD

Sedation
Danielle Devereaux, MD
Attending Physician
Departments of Emergency Medicine
   & Pediatrics
Prince George Hospital Center
Cheverly, MD

Joey M. Scollan, DO
Attending Physician
Departments of Emergency Medicine
   & Pediatrics
Elliot Hospital
Manchester, NH

SINGLE-DOSE PRESSORS
James Lantry, MD
Associate Professor
Departments of Emergency Medicine &
   Critical Care Medicine
San Antonio Military Medical Complex
San Antonio, TX

PROTOCOLS
Post-Arrest Hypothermia
Kami M. Hu, MD
Chief Resident
Emergency Medicine & Internal
   Medicine Combined Residency
University of Maryland Medical Center
Baltimore, MD

Daniel Boutsikaris, MD
Attending Physician
Departments of Emergency Medicine &
   Critical Care Program
Rutgers-Robert Wood Johnson
   University Hospital
New Brunswick, NJ

Table of Contents

■ Pulmonary

■ Sepsis

■ Toxicology

■ Pediatrics

■ Miscellaneous

Vasoactive Agent Overview

Agent	Mechanism	Effects	Clinical Usage	General Dosing Range
Dobutamine *Inotrope*	$\uparrow\beta_1$ $\uparrow\beta_2$	Increases CO, SV	Cardiogenic shock Septic shock	2.5-20 mcg/kg/min
Dopamine *Vasopressor* *Inotrope*	DA at low doses $\uparrow\alpha_1$ $\uparrow\alpha_2$ $\uparrow\beta_1$	Increases CO Vasoconstriction at higher doses	Septic shock Cardiogenic shock Neurogenic shock	5-20 mcg/kg/min
Dopexamine *Inotrope*	$\uparrow\beta_2 >> \uparrow\beta_1$ DA	Increases CO Mild afterload reduction	Low CO cardiogenic or septic shock	0.5-6 mcg/kg/min
Epinephrine *Vasopressor* *Inotrope*	$\uparrow\alpha_1$ $\uparrow\alpha_2$ $\uparrow\beta_1$ $\uparrow\beta_2$	Increases HR, SV, CO Vasoconstriction at higher doses	Septic shock Low-output cardiogenic shock Anaphylactic shock	0.05-0.5 mcg/kg/min *(No true max, but reports of dosing as high as 5 mcg/kg/min)*
Isoproterenol *Chronotrope*	$\uparrow\beta_1$ $\uparrow\beta_2$	Decreases SVR Increases CO HR >> SV	Temporary support for hemodynamically unstable bradycardias refractory to atropine	0.5-5 mcg/min
Milrinone *Inotrope*	Inhibits PDE $\uparrow$ Intracellular Ca^{2+} causing $\uparrow$ cAMP	Increases diastolic relaxation, CO, vasodilation	Low CO cardiogenic or septic shock	0.375-0.75 mcg/kg/min
Norepinephrine *Vasopressor* *Inotrope*	α_1 +/- α_2 $\uparrow\beta_1$ $\uparrow\beta_2$	Increased vaso-constriction and mild increase in cardiac output	Septic shock Cardiogenic shock	0.05-0.5 mcg/kg/min *(No true max, but reports of dosing as high as 5 mcg/kg/min)*
Phenylephrine *Vasopressor*	$\uparrow\alpha_1$	Increases SVR Decreases CO at high doses	Vasodilatory shock Procedural hypotension	2-10 mcg/kg bolus **THEN** 1-5 mcg/kg/min
Vasopressin *Vasopressor*	Increases levels of IP_3 and DAG, which cause an $\uparrow$ in intracellular Ca^{2+}	Increases peripheral vasoconstriction	Septic shock (high cardiac output shock)	0.04-0.1 units/min

HR = Heart rate
SV = Stroke volume

SVR = Systemic vascular resistance
CO = Cardiac output

2015 EMRA PressorDex

Pressor

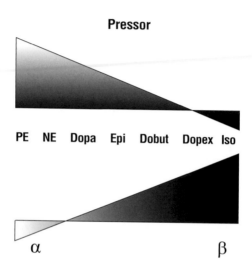

Hollenberg SM. Vasoactive drugs in circulatory shock. *Am J Respir Crit Care Med* 2011;183:847-55.

Indications

- Rapid-sequence induction (RSI): quick induction of deep sedation
- Procedural sedation: moderate sedation, rapid onset/offset, patient maintains own airway
- Intermittent bolus sedation: initiate post-intubation; use continuous sedation if multiple boluses are needed.
- Continuous sedation: sedation degree depends on clinical goals; initiate post-intubation.

Agent	Pharmaco-kinetics[1]	Indication	Dose	Warnings/Special uses
Benzodiazepines				
Lorazepam (Ativan)	Onset: 5-20 min Duration: 6-8 hrs Half-life: 8-15 hrs	RSI (not 1st line)	N/A	Slower onset but longer acting; effective anxiolytic; watch for met. Acidosis and acute kidney failure due to propylene glycol diluent, follow Osmol gap for surveillance; over-sedation risk with rapid titration.
		Proc. sedation	N/A	
		Int. sedation	1-4 mg	
		Cont. sedation	1-4 mg bolus 0.01-0.1 mg/kg/hr (titrate q1 hr)	
Midazolam (Versed)	Onset: 60-90 sec Duration: 2-4 hrs Half-life: 1-4 hrs	RSI	0.1-0.3 mg/kg (2nd line agent)	IM or IV, often used with fentanyl; short duration, but with long-term use, has long half-life; has CYP 3A4 interactions.
		Proc. sedation	0.05 mg/kg (titrate q3 min)	
		Int. sedation	1-5 mg bolus	
		Cont. sedation	0.04-0.2 mg/kg/hr (titrate q1 hr)	
Sedative-Hypnotics				
Propofol (Diprivan)	Onset: <1 min Duration: 3-10 min Half-life: 5-10 min	RSI	2 mg/kg	Can ↓ BP and HR; antiepileptic; prolonged use or high doses ↑ risk of propofol infusion syndrome; monitor triglycerides (TG), amylase/lipase; egg/soybean allergy CI, peanut allergy CI with propofol, safe in renal or hepatic failure.
		Proc. sedation	1 mg/kg (repeat 0.5 mg/kg q5 min)	
		Cont. sedation	5-80 mcg/kg/min (titrate q10 min)	

	Sedative-Hypnotics *continued*			
Agent	**Pharmaco-kinetics[1]**	**Indication**	**Dose[2,3]**	**Warnings/Special Uses**
Etomidate (Amidate)	Onset: <1 min Duration: 3-5 min Half-life: 3-12 min	RSI	0.3 mg/kg (1-time dose)	May cause myoclonus, hemodynamically (HD) stable and rapid onset; can suppress adrenals x24 hrs (of controversial significance).
		Proc. sedation	0.1-0.2 mg/kg (2nd line, 1-time dose)	
		Cont. sedation	N/A	
Dexme-detomidine (Precedex)	Onset: 5-30 min Duration:1-2 hrs Half-life: 2 hrs	RSI	N/A	Only sedative approved for non-intubated pts, may still lose airway reflexes; minimal respiratory depression; ↓BP, ↓HR; ↑BP with large/loading doses, anxiolytic/some analgesic effects; α_2-agonist causing sympatholysis (e.g., bradycardia).
		Proc. sedation	0.5-1 mcg/kg over 10 min	
		Cont. sedation	0.2-1.5 mcg/kg/hr (titrate q1 hr)	

	Dissociatives			
Ketamine	Onset: <1 min Duration: 30-45 min Half-life: 5-15 min	RSI	1-2 mg/kg IV or 4-10 mg/kg IM	May ↑ ICP and BP; maintains resp drive, good for awake intubation; may ↓ bronchospasm; can cause emergence reaction, nausea, laryngospasm, or hypersalivation (may need succinylcholine, glycopyrrolate or atropine); caution in severe heart failure.
		Proc. sedation	1 mg/kg (repeat 1 mg/kg q10 min)	
		Cont. sedation	0.5-1 mg/kg/hr (2nd line agent)	

	Opiates			
Morphine	Onset: <1 min Duration: 2-4 hrs Half-life: 2-3 hrs	Analgesia	0.5-10 mg bolus 0.5-80 mg/hr (titrate q1 hr)	Can cause hypotension, histamine release; tolerance develops with chronic use.
Fentanyl	Onset: <30 sec Duration: 30-60 min Half-life: 2-4 hrs	Analgesia, sedation	1-3 mcg/kg bolus 25-250 mcg/hr (titrate q20 min)	More HD stable; faster acting; tolerance develops with chronic use; accumulates in liver, less hypotension, can cause ACS* with high dose, tx with succinylcholine.

Opiates *continued*				
Agent	**Pharmaco-kinetics[1]**	**Indication**	**Dose[2,3]**	**Warnings/Special Uses**
Remifentanil	Onset: <1 min Duration: 3-10 in Half-life: 3-10 in	Analgesia, sedation	1-1.5 mcg/kg bolus 0.25-0.5 mcg/kg/min (titrate q5 min). *Ideal* body weight (IBW) if obese.	Ultra-short acting; allows for frequent neurologic exams, safe in renal and hepatic failure.

Onset and duration differ for single doses and repeated doses.
Doses are for IV route unless specified otherwise.
Consider adjusted doses for obesity and end-organ compromise.

Note: See Appendix 1 for commonly used sedation scales.

Reversal Agents

- Naloxone (opioids): Start with 0.4 mg IV bolus and titrate with incremental doses up to 2 mg total (use 1-2 mL of 1:10 diluted solution per bolus). Prepare this solution by mixing naloxone 0.4 mg/1 ml with 9 ml NSS for final concentration of 0.04 mg/ml. May be given IM or SC; also inhalation via nebulization.
- Flumazenil (benzodiazepines):
  - For acute overdose, start with 0.2 mg over 30 sec, followed by 0.3 mg over 30 sec **THEN** subsequent doses of 0.5 mg over 30 sec (q1 min) up to 5 mg.
  - For reversal of procedural sedation, start with 0.2 mg over 15 sec **THEN** 0.2 mg q1 min x 4 doses as needed.
  - Rarely used in chronic benzodiazepine users due to risk of inducing intractable seizures; used primarily in procedural sedation reversal.

Additional therapeutic options and considerations

- Ketofol (combination ketamine-propofol): Comparison data equivocal at this time. May provide select reduced side effect profile and reduction in re-dosing requirements.
  - Suggested mixing at 1:1 ratio.
  - Initial bolus 0.5 mg/kg each ketamine and propofol with PRN boluses of 0.5 mg/kg of the mixture.
    - Safety issues with its use are recognized: sterility measures upon mixing not met; and accurate labels, including concentration of each drug and expiration dating, not applied, result in contamination and administration errors, respectively; compatibility data are also lacking.

PEARLS

→ Always give sedation BEFORE paralysis.
→ Have airway backup equipment ready for all procedural sedation.
→ Consider ketamine for difficult sedations or refractory agitation.
→ Hold continuous sedation on a regular basis (i.e., "sedation vacation" or "spontaneous awakening trials") and attempt weaning of sedation dose daily.
→ Check if analgesia requirements are being met before increasing sedation.
→ Richmond Agitation-Sedation Scale (RASS) or Riker Sedation-Agitation Scale (SAS) should be used over physiologic measure of brain fx (auditory evoked potential, bispectral index, etc.).

Indications

- Optimize intubation conditions.
- Facilitate ventilator synchrony and decrease oxygen consumption in acute respiratory distress syndrome or status asthmaticus.
- Adjunct in management of intracranial or intra-abdominal hypertension.
- Prevent shivering during targeted temperature management after cardiac arrest.

Treatment: Common Agents for Rapid-Sequence Intubation

Agent	Type of Blockade	Onset	Duration	Dose	Elimination
Succinylcholine	Depolarizing	Rapid (45-60 sec)	5-10 min	Bolus: 1-1.5 mg/kg Infusion: None	Rapidly cleared by plasma cholinesterases
Rocuronium	Non-depolarizing	Rapid (1-2 min)	30-60 min	Bolus: 0.6-1.2 mg/kg	Hepatobiliary and renal clearance

Treatment: Common Agents for Continuous Paralysis

Agent	Type of Blockade	Onset	Duration	Dose	Elimination
Vecuronium	Non-depolarizing	Moderate (2-4 min)	30-60 min	Bolus: 0.1-0.2 mg/kg Infusion: 0.8-1.2 mcg/kg/min	Hepatobiliary and renal clearance
Cisatracurium	Non-depolarizing	Slow (3-5 min)	30-60 min	Bolus: 0.1-0.2 mg/kg Infusion: 0.5-10 mcg/kg/min	Hofmann elimination, so preferred in organ dysfunction

Adverse effects with succinylcholine

- Bradycardia (more common in pediatric patients or with repeat dosing).
- Malignant hyperthermia
- Hyperkalemia (common in chronic neuromuscular disease, subacute or chronic burns, prolonged immobilization or paralysis >72 hrs, chronic renal failure).
- Long-acting effect in patients with genetic pseudocholinesterase deficiency or after plasmapheresis.

Other agents

- Long-acting, non-depolarizing agents such as pancuronium, D-tubocurarine, and pipecuronium are used less commonly; intermediate-acting agents include atracurium and mivacurium.
- **Anticholinesterases** such as **neostigmine** help overcome competitive neuromuscular blockers. Cholinergic side effects may occur; coadminister with glycopyrrolate or atropine.
- **Sugammadex** encapsulates and binds rocuronium and vecuronium, reversing blockade; used in Europe (not FDA-approved).

PEARLS

→ Choice of agent is based on onset, desired duration of action, clearance, and side effects.
→ Critical to ensure adequate sedation and analgesia for the duration of paralysis.
→ Effects of blockade are potentiated by hypokalemia, acidosis, hypocalcemia, hypermagnesemia, furosemide, verapamil, and aminoglycoside antibiotics.
→ Hypothermia may prolong the duration of action of paralytics.
→ A peripheral nerve stimulator may be used to assess degree of neuromuscular blockade.
→ Consider using ideal body weight (IBW) for the morbidly obese patient.

ABDOMINAL AORTIC ANEURYSM (AAA) RUPTURE
Hemorrhagic/Hypovolemic Shock

Differential Diagnosis

- Renal colic
- Cholecystitis
- GI hemorrhage
- Gastritis
- Acute myocardial infarction
- Diverticulitis
- Peptic ulcer disease
- Aortic dissection
- Perforated viscus
- Pancreatitis
- Ischemic bowel
- Idiopathic back pain

Treatment

Aggressive stabilization and emergent vascular surgery consultation is recommended.

- **Resuscitation**
  - Two large-bore peripheral or central venous access
  - 0.9% NS bolus or O negative blood; activate massive transfusion protocol.
- **Vasopressors**
  May be necessary to maintain adequate end-organ perfusion.
  Permissive hypotension (systolic BP 60-70) can prevent further tearing of aorta and additional blood loss.
  - Norepinephrine
    - Infusion: 0.05 mcg/kg/min IV, titrate by 0.02 mcg/kg/min q5 min
    - Dose range: 0.05-0.5 mcg/kg/min; Onset: 1-2 min; Duration: 1-2 min
    - No true max, but consider using additional agents if patient is unresponsive to higher doses.
  - Phenylephrine (Neo-synephrine)
    - Infusion: 100-180 mcg/min, titrate by 25 mcg/min q10 min
    - Weight-based dosing: 0.5 mcg/kg/min, titrate to response
    - Dose range: 0.5-9 mcg/kg/min; Onset: 1-2 min; Duration: 15-20 min
  - Dopamine
    - Infusion: 5 mcg/kg/min, titrate by 5 mcg/kg/min q10 min
    - Max dose: 50 mcg/kg/min; Onset: 5 min; Duration: <10 min
    - Note: dose >10-20 mcg/kg/min may increase risk of tachyarrhythmia and increase sheer stress on the aortic wall.

PEARLS

→ Classic presentation: smoker >60 with hypertension, and the triad of severe pain, hypotension and a pulsatile mass or known AAA.

→ "Atypical is typical": may present as abdominal or flank pain (75%), nausea or vomiting (20%), syncope (10-30%), hematuria, groin pain.

→ Ultrasound is highly sensitive in detecting aortic dilation, but should not delay other necessary imaging (CT) or emergency surgery.

→ FAST exam often negative; 80% of ruptures bleed into retroperitoneum.

→ AAA is more common in men; however, the rate of growth and risk of rupture is higher in women.

→ Bradycardia may be a sign of intraperitoneal blood.

→ Consider mycotic aneurysm in the above patient with a fever.

ACUTE CORONARY SYNDROME

ST-segment elevation MI (STEMI)

- *Reperfusion therapy*
  - Percutaneous intervention (PCI) with balloon angioplasty/stenting is *preferred*.
  - Thrombolytics (if no catheterization lab is available or nearby administer within 30 minutes of hospital arrival)
    - Tissue plasminogen activator (t-PA)
      - Alteplase
        - Initial dose: 15 mg IV push over 1-2 min
        - Second dose: 0.75 mg/kg IV over 30 min, max dose 50 mg
        - Third dose: 0.5 mg/kg IV over 60 min, max dose 35 mg
      - Reteplase
        - Initial dose: 10 units IV push over 2 min
        - Second dose: 10 units IV push over 2 min, 30 min after first bolus
    - Tenecteplase: 30-50 mg IV push over 5 sec (based on body weight)
- *Also incorporate additional therapies used for NSTEMI/UA (see below).*
- *See Table 1 for contraindications.*

Table 1: Contraindications to Thrombolytics in STEMI	
Absolute contraindications	
• Any prior ICH • Known structural cerebral vascular lesion (e.g., AVM) • Known malignant intracranial neoplasm (primary or metastatic) • Severe, uncontrolled HTN unresponsive to therapy (SBP >180 mmHg or DBP >110 mmHg)†	• Intracranial/spinal surgery within 2 months • Suspected aortic dissection • Active bleeding or bleeding diathesis (excluding menses) • Significant closed head or facial trauma within 3 months • Streptokinase (within 6 months)
Relative contraindications	
• History of chronic severe, poorly controlled hypertension • History of prior ischemic stroke greater than 3 months, dementia, or known intracranial pathology not covered in contraindications • Traumatic or prolonged (>10 min) CPR • Major surgery (<3 weeks) • Recent (within 2 to 4 weeks) internal bleeding • Noncompressible vascular punctures • Pregnancy • Active peptic ulcer • Current use of anticoagulants (the higher the INR, the higher the risk of bleeding)	

Note: There is no absolute contraindication for any patient in cardiac arrest.

Non-ST segment elevated MI (NSTEMI)/unstable angina (UA)

- *Increase myocardial oxygenation/reduce angina.*
  - Nitroglycerin
    - Sublingual: 1 spray or tablet (400 mcg) q5 min x 3
    - Infusion: 10 mcg/min IV, titrate by 5 mcg/min q3-5 min to 20 mcg/min
      - If no response at 20 mcg/min, titrate by 10-20 mcg/min q3-5 min.
    - Max: 200 mcg/min; Onset: immediate; Duration: 3-5 min
      - Avoid if HR <60 bpm, HR >100 bpm in absence of heart failure, hypotension (SBP <90 mmHg or >/= 30 mmHg drop from baseline), PDE-5 inhibitors (e.g., sildenafil) used, or pericarditis.
      - Beware of precipitous BP drop with RV infarction.
- *Reduce thrombus propagation.*
  - Antiplatelet therapy
    - Aspirin: 162-325 mg PO
    - *Consider* (consult with cardiologist prior to administration):
      - Thienopyridine-class inhibitor
        - Clopidogrel: 300-600 mg PO, followed by 75 mg PO qday
        - Prasugrel: 60 mg PO, followed by 10 mg PO qday
          - Maintenance dose reduction to 5 mg PO daily <60 kg
          - Not recommended in patients >/= 75 years of age
        - Ticagrelor: 180 mg PO, followed by 90 mg PO bid
      - Glycoprotein IIb/IIIa inhibitors *(in conjunction with UFH or bivalirudin)*
        - Eptifibatide
          - Loading dose: 180 mcg/kg IV (max 22.6 mg)
          - Infusion (maintenance): 2 mcg/kg/min until hospital discharge (max 15 mg/hour)
          - PCI candidate: repeat bolus 180 mcg/kg IV (max 22.6 mg), 10 min after first bolus, **THEN** 2 mcg/kg/min (max 15 mg/hour) for 18-24 hrs after procedure
          - Renal dose adjustment for patients with creatinine clearance <50 mL/min
            - Loading dose: 180 mcg/kg IV bolus (max 22.6 mg)
            - Infusion (maintenance): 1 mcg/kg/min (max 7.5 mg/hr)
        - Abciximab *(preferred agent in renal dysfunction)*
          - Loading dose: 0.25 mg/kg IV
          - Infusion (maintenance): 10 mcg/min IV for 18-24 hrs
          - PCI candidate infusion: 0.125 mcg/kg/min IV for 12 hrs (max 10 mcg/min)
        - Tirofiban
          - Loading dose: 25 mg/kg IV
          - Infusion (maintenance): 0.15 mcg/kg/min IV for 18-24 hrs
          - Renal dose adjustment: CrCl <60 ml/min, reduce maintenance dose to 0.075 mg/kg/min

- Anticoagulants
    - Unfractionated heparin: aPTT goal of 1.5 – 2 x control (approx. 50-70s) for 48 hrs or until revascularization
        - Loading dose: 60 units/kg IV (max 5000 units)
        - Infusion: 12 units/kg/hr (max 1000 units/hr)
    - Low-molecular-weight heparin (LMWH)
        - Enoxaparin: 1 mg/kg subcut q12 hrs
        - *If candidate for PCI or thrombolysis: 30 mg IV push prior to procedure*
            - *If patient is >75 y/o, consider reducing dose to 0.75 mg/kg subcut q12hrs (max dose 75 mg for first 2 doses), and do not give IV push dose of enoxaparin.*
    - Bivalirudin *(preferred over UFH in high risk of bleeding)*
        - Loading dose: 0.75 mg/kg
        - Infusion (maintenance): 1.75 mg/kg/hr
        - Renal dose adjustment for patients with creatinine clearance <30 mL/min
            - Infusion (maintenance): 1 mcg/kg/hr
    - Fondaparinux *(not recommended as sole anticoagulant for PCI)*
        - Loading dose: 2.5 mg/kg IV push
        - Maintenance: 2.5 mg/kg subcut qday
        - Contraindicated in patients with CrCl <30 ml/min

ACS with cardiogenic shock (CS)
Emergent revascularization with PCI or CABG; fibrinolytic therapy considered 2nd line.
Blood pressure support
- *Consider* intra-aortic balloon pump counterpulsation (IABP) or left ventricular assist devices.
- Vasopressors/inotropes: goal MAP >65 mmHg
    - Norepinephrine
        - Infusion: 0.05 mcg/kg/min IV, titrate by 0.02 mcg/kg/min q5 min
        - Dose range: 0.05-0.5 mcg/kg/min; Onset: 1-2 min; Duration: 1-2 min
        - No true max, but consider using additional agents if patient is unresponsive to higher doses.
    - Isoproterenol: β_1/β_2 agonist for bradycardic CS
        - Loading dose: 0.02-0.06 mg IV
            - Bolus dose reserved for heart block, not CS.
        - Infusion: 5 mcg/min IV, titrate to max of 20 mcg/min for goal HR of 60 bpm
    - Dobutamine:
        - Infusion: 2.5 mcg/kg/min IV, **THEN** titrate by 2.5 mcg/kg/min q10 min
        - Max: 20 mcg/kg/min; Onset: 1-2 min; Duration: 10 min
    - Dobutamine:
        - Infusion: 5-10 mcg/kg/min IV, **THEN** titrate by 1-4 mcg/kg/min q10-30 min
        - Max: 50 mcg/kg/min; Onset: 5 min; Duration: 10 min

→ Use bedside ultrasound to rule out other causes of CS and to guide therapy.
→ All ACS patients should receive β-blockers within 24 hrs, not emergently in the ED.
→ Treat symptomatic cocaine-induced ACS with benzodiazepines; phentolamine may be considered if blood pressure is severely elevated.
→ PCI: In general, should be performed within <90 min of arrival in ED.
→ Consider urgent PCI in symptomatic NSTEMI/UA refractory to aggressive medical therapy.
→ Transcutaneous/transvenous pacing is recommended for shock secondary to bradycardia (e.g., RV infarction).
→ Current guidelines recommend use of IABP for CS refractory to pharmacological therapy, despite lack of evidence for decreased morbidity/mortality (IABP-SHOCK II).

AORTIC DISSECTION

Treatment Goals

- Immediate BP goal: SBP 100-120 mmHg (or MAP 60-75) **PLUS** HR 60-70 bpm
- **Type A dissection:** Involvement of ascending aorta proximal to ligamentum arteriosum
- **Type B dissection:** Involvement of the aorta distal to ligamentum arteriosum

Heart rate control

- Esmolol: negative inotrope/chronotrope (β-blocker)
  - Loading dose: 500 mcg/kg IV bolus over 1 min (can repeat loading dose once)
  - Infusion: 50 mcg/kg/min, titrate by 50 mcg/kg/min q4 min
  - Max: 300 mcg/kg/min; Onset: 1-2 min; Duration: 10-30 min
- Diltiazem: negative inotrope/chronotrope and arterial vasodilator
  - Loading dose: 0.25 mg/kg IV over 2 min (average adult dose = 20 mg)
  - Infusion: 5 mg/hr, titrate by 5 mg/hr q15 min
  - Max: 15 mg/hr; Onset: 3 min; Duration: 1-10 hrs

Blood pressure control

- Nicardipine: pure arterial vasodilator
  - Infusion: 5 mg/hr, titrate by 2.5 mg/hr q5 min
  - Max: 15 mg/hr; Onset: 5-15 min; Duration: 4-6 hrs
- Labetalol: negative inotrope and arterial vasodilator
  - Loading dose: 20 mg IV over 2 min
  - Infusion: 2-8 mg/min, titrate by 0.5 mg/min q10 min
  - Max: 8 mg/min; Onset: 2-5 min; Duration 2-4 hrs
    - Note: Consider alternative agents if BP unresponsive to high doses.
- Nitroprusside: venous and arterial vasodilator
  - Infusion: 0.25-0.3 mcg/kg/min, titrate by 0.5 mcg/kg/min q2 min
  - Max: 10 mcg/kg/min; Onset: 1-2 min; Duration: 10 min
  - Note: Doses >/= 2 mcg/kg/min are associated with higher risk of cyanide toxicity. If no response seen after giving 10 mcg/kg/min for 10 minutes, discontinue nitroprusside and use alternative agent.

- Fenoldopam: D1 receptor agonist, peripheral vasodilator
  - Infusion: 0.03-0.1 mcg/kg/min, titrate by 0.05-0.1 mcg/kg/min q15 min
  - Max: 1.6 mcg/kg/min; Onset: 15 min; Duration: 1-4 hrs

PEARLS

→ Consider dissection in the setting of an abnormal neurologic exam that is inconsistent with a cerebral distribution.

→ Always start β-blocker (or other negative inotropes if β-blockers contraindicated) before antihypertensive agent to prevent reflex tachycardia.

→ Monitor patients for end-organ malperfusion (e.g., mesenteric ischemia).

→ Consider fenoldopam when renal insufficiency present or renal artery involvement.

→ Consider TEE as initial diagnostic modality.

→ Pulse deficit on exam present in <20% of patients with aortic dissection.

ATRIAL FIBRILLATION/ATRIAL FLUTTER WITH RVR
Cardiogenic Shock

Differential Diagnosis

- Rapid, narrow complex, irregular rhythm
  - Ddx: Atrial fibrillation with RVR; atrial flutter with variable conduction; multifocal atrial tachycardia
  - Atrial fibrillation with pre-excitation (WPW) should be considered with **wide-complex irregular rhythm**; avoid AV nodal blocking agents, which can cause ventricular tachycardia and ventricular fibrillation.

Treatment

Unstable: myocardial ischemia, symptomatic hypotension, ischemic chest pain, acute heart failure, altered mental status

- *Synchronized electrical cardioversion:*
  - Administer sedatives and analgesics prior to cardioversion.
  - Start with 120-200J biphasic.
  - Start with 200J monophasic.
    - Escalate energy levels with subsequent shocks as needed.
    - Atrial flutter may only require 50J-100J initially.

Stable – Goal Heart Rate <110 beats/min

- Diltiazem
  - Initial dose: 10 mg to 20 mg IV bolus (0.25 mg/kg dose over 2 min)
  - 2nd dose: 15 mg to 25 mg IV bolus (0.35 mg/kg), 15 min later PRN
  - Infusion: 5 mg/hr, titrate by 5 mg/hr q15 min
  - Max: 15 mg/hr; Onset: 3 min; Duration: 1-3 hr (bolus); 1-10 hrs (infusion, prolonged if infusion >24 hrs)

- Metoprolol
  - Initial dose: 2.5-5 mg IV bolus over 1-2 min
  - May repeat dose every 5 min up to 15 mg total over 10- to 15-minute interval.
  - Maintenance: 25 mg PO every 12 hrs **OR** atenolol 25 mg PO once daily
  - Onset: 5 minutes; Peak effect: 20 minutes; Duration: 5-8 hours
- Esmolol
  - Loading dose: 500 mcg/kg IV bolus over 1 min (can repeat loading dose twice)
  - Infusion: 50 mcg/kg/min, titrate by 50 mcg/kg/min every 5 min
  - Max: 200 mcg/kg/min; Onset: 1-2 min; Duration 10-30 min
- *Digoxin: Consider in patients with advanced heart failure or moderate hypotension, and when adequate rate control cannot be achieved with calcium channel blockers and β-blockers.*
  - Loading dose: 250 mcg q2 hrs IV or PO (up to max dose of 1.5 mg)
    - Total combined loading dose is typically 750 mcg to 1 mg.
  - Maintenance: 125 to 375 mcg IV/PO once daily
  - Onset: >1 hour; Peak effect: 1-6 hours; Duration 3-4 days
- Amiodarone: *Consider in patients with heart failure or hypotension, and when adequate rate control cannot be achieved with calcium channel blockers and β-blockers.*
  - Loading: 150 mg IV bolus, may repeat 150 mg IV
  - Infusion: 1 mg/min for 6 hrs, **THEN** 0.5 mg/min

PEARLS

→ Evaluate patient for underlying cause(s) of dysrhythmia (electrolytes, dehydration, etc.) and reverse.

→ Use caution in patients with severe or decompensated heart failure when giving negative inotropes (especially calcium channel blockers).

→ Diltiazem may cause hypotension. Consider pre-treatment with calcium gluconate 1-2 grams IV, and consider smaller aliquots of 5 mg at a time if hypotension is a concern.

→ Thromboembolism is a risk with conversion of chronic A-fib to sinus rhythm, start heparin bolus and infusion in patients with A-fib and A-flutter >48 hrs requiring emergent cardioversion.

→ Consider procainamide for rapid A-fib with pre-excitation not requiring emergent cardioversion (*see SVT+AV Node Re-entry/Pre-excitation in the Supraventricular Tachycardia chapter*).

CONGESTIVE HEART FAILURE
Cardiogenic Shock

Treatment

If SBP >100 mmHg without signs of shock:

- Diuresis if evidence of pulmonary vascular congestion.
    - Furosemide
        - Initial dose: 40 mg IV or same mg home oral dose given as IV; increase by 20 mg/dose after 1-2 hours as needed.
            - Repeat dose q6-24 hrs for urine output (UOP) goal >0.5 ml/kg/hr, max 160 mg/dose
        - Infusion:
            - Initial dose: 40 mg IV bolus, **THEN** 10-40 mg/hr
            - Goal: UOP >0.5 mL/kg/hr; check BMP q6 hrs
    - Bumetanide
        - Initial dose: 0.5-1 mg IV; may repeat dose in 2 to 3 hrs; max 10 mg/day
        - Infusion: Initial 1 mg IV bolus, **THEN** 0.5-2 mg/hr
- Congestive symptoms refractory to diuresis
    - Nitroglycerin (NTG)
        - Sublingual: 1 spray or 0.4 mg tablet (400 mcg) q5 min
        - Loading dose (if not given orally): 50-100 mcg/min for 1-5 minutes
        - Infusion: 50-200 mcg/min, titrate by 40 mcg/min q3-5 min
        - Max: 200 mcg/min; Onset: 2-5 min; Duration: 3-5 min
            - If minimal symptoms, can use topical NTG, 0.5-1 inch q6 hrs
            - Avoid if evidence of right ventricular MI, HR <60 bpm, PDE-5 inhibitors (e.g., sildenafil) used, or pericarditis present.
    - Captopril
        - Initial dose: 12.5 mg sublingual x 1
        - Dose range: 12.5-50 mg PO tid
- **If patient shows signs of shock and MAP >65 mmHg or SBP >90 mmHg, start inotropic therapy for a goal cardiac index (CI) >2.5 L/min/m^2, ScVO2 >70%.**
    - Dobutamine
        - Infusion: 2.5 mcg/kg/min IV, titrate by 2.5 mcg/kg/min q10 min
        - Max: 20 mcg/kg/min; Onset: 1-2 min; Duration: 10 min
    - Milrinone
        - Loading dose: 50 mcg/kg IV over 10 min (consider omitting due to potential decrease in BP)
        - Infusion: 0.375 mcg/kg/min IV, titrate by 0.005 mcg/kg/min q5-10 min
        - Max: 0.75 mcg/kg/min; Onset: 5-15 min; Duration: 3-5 hrs
        - *Note: Duration of action prolonged when renal insufficiency present.*

- **If signs of shock and MAP <65 mmHg, initiate vasopressor therapy.**
  - Norepinephrine
    - Infusion: 0.05 mcg/kg/min IV, titrate by 0.02 mcg/kg/min q5 min
    - Dose range: 0.05-0.5 mcg/kg/min; Onset: 1-2 min; Duration: 1-2 min
    - No true max, but consider using additional agents if patient is unresponsive to higher doses.
  - Epinephrine
    - Infusion: 1-2 mcg/min IV, titrate by 1 mcg/min q10 min
    - Dose range: 0.05-0.5 mcg/kg/min; Onset: 1-2 min
    - *In addition to vasopressor effect, offers inotropic support in patients with low cardiac index.*
  - Dopamine
    - Infusion: 5 mcg/kg/min IV, titrate by 5 mcg/kg/min q10 min
    - Max: 50 mcg/kg/min; Onset: 5 min; Duration: <10 min
      - Note: dose >20 mcg/kg/min may not benefit BP and **may increase risk of tachydysrhythmia**.

Additional therapeutic options and considerations

- Noninvasive positive pressure ventilation (NIPPV) should be considered first-line therapy in patients with acute CHF; decreases intubation and mortality.
- Non-pharmacologic therapy: Consider intra-aortic balloon pump or consultation for left ventricular assist device in refractory cases.

PEARLS

→ Rapid bedside echocardiogram can help differentiate common causes, including systolic or diastolic dysfunction, acute MI, or valvular dysfunction.

→ Patients presenting with pulmonary vascular congestion may actually be intravascularly depleted. Therapy in this population should focus on redistribution of the pulmonary congestion with preload reduction (e.g., NIPPV, NTG), afterload reduction (e.g., NIPPV, ACE-I), and potentially inotropic support.

→ Consider ultrafiltration if patient is refractory to aggressive diuretic therapy.

→ Morphine administration is associated with an increased need for intubation and independently predicts increased mortality, so avoid its use for acute CHF.

HYPERTENSIVE EMERGENCY (ESSENTIAL)

Indication

Severe hypertension (i.e., systolic blood pressure >160 mmHg and/or diastolic blood pressure >110 mmHg) *plus* end-organ dysfunction, which may include the following:

- Intracerebral hemorrhage
- Myocardial ischemia
- Acute renal failure
- Pulmonary edema
- Aortic dissection

Treatment

Target blood pressure should be a MAP decrease of 20-25% within 24 hours.

- Clevidipine (if available): pure arterial vasodilator
  - Infusion: 1 mg/hr *THEN* double rate q90 sec until close to goal; titrate by 1-2 mg/hr q5-10 min PRN
  - Max: 21 mg/hr; Onset: 2-4 min; Duration: 5-15 min
- Nicardipine: pure arterial vasodilator
  - Infusion: 5 mg/hr, titrate by 2.5 mg/hr q5 min
  - Max: 15 mg/hr; Onset: 5-15 min; Duration: 4-6 hrs
- Labetalol
  - Loading dose: 20 mg IV, double dose at 10-min intervals to max of 300 mg
  - Infusion: 2-8 mg/min, titrate by 0.5 mg/min q10 min
  - Max: 8 mg/min; Onset: 2-5 min; Duration: 2-4 hrs
    - *Note: Consider alternative agents if patient remains on high dose of labetalol.*
- Nitroglycerin: pure venous vasodilator *(consider for patients with CHF)*
  - Loading dose: 50-100 mcg/min for 1-5 min
  - Infusion: 50-200 mcg/min, titrate by 40 mcg/min q3-5 min
  - Max: 200 mcg/min; Onset: 2-5 min; Duration 3-5 minutes
    - Avoid if HR <60 bpm, PDE-5 inhibitors (e.g., sildenafil) are used, or pericarditis is present.
- Nitroprusside: arterial and venous vasodilator *(last resort)*
  - Infusion: 0.25-0.5 mcg/kg/min IV, titrate by 0.25-0.5 mcg/kg/min q2-3 min
  - Max: 8-10 mcg/kg/min; Onset: 1-2 min; Duration: 1-10 min
  - Note: Doses >2 mcg/kg/min for prolonged period is associated with increased risk of cyanide toxicity. If BP not controlled with 10 mcg/kg/min for 10 minutes, discontinue nitroprusside and use alternative therapy.
- Fenoldopam (D_1 receptor agonist); *consider in patients with renal insufficiency*
  - Infusion: 0.05 mcg/kg/min, titrate by 0.05-0.1 mcg/kg/min q15 min
  - Max: 1.6 mcg/kg/min; Onset: 4 min; Duration: <10 min

→ Consider arterial line placement during medication titration for precise monitoring.
→ Avoid overzealous correction, as this can lead to organ hypoperfusion. Monitor for worsening mental status, pulmonary edema, and chest pain.
→ Avoid bolus-dose agents (e.g., hydralazine, enalapril) due to unpredictable absorption, efficacy, and duration of action.
→ Blood pressure and blood flow are not synonymous. Patients are often hypovolemic due to prolonged pressure-natriuresis, so IV fluid resuscitation is often required.

SUPRAVENTRICULAR TACHYCARDIA (SVT)
Cardiogenic Shock

Treatment
Unstable: myocardial ischemia, symptomatic hypotension, angina, acute heart failure, altered mental status
- *Synchronized cardioversion:*
  - Administer sedatives and analgesics prior to cardioversion.
  - Start with 120-200J biphasic.
  - Start with 200J monophasic.
    - Escalate energy levels with subsequent shocks as needed.

Stable SVT
First-line recommendations
- Vagal maneuvers
- Adenosine
  - Initial dose: 6 mg IV fast push, followed by 20 mL rapid saline push
  - 2nd dose: 12 mg IV fast push; if unsuccessful, may repeat 12 mg IV fast push
    - Reduce to 3 mg: AV nodal blocking is enhanced in central line usage, heart transplants, and usage of dipyridamole or carbamazepine.
    - Increase to 12 mg IV push: AV nodal blocking is antagonized by methylxanthines such as caffeine and theophylline; larger doses may be required and may not work at all.
    - Use caution in asthmatic patients – may cause bronchoconstriction and bronchospasm.
    - AV nodal blocker can cause asystole or ventricular fibrillation for AVNRT; keep defibrillation equipment nearby.
- Calcium channel blockers (CCB) can be used as first- or second-line treatment.
  - Verapamil
    - Initial dose: 0.075 mg/kg IV (usually 5 mg) over 2 min
    - 2nd dose: 0.15 mg/kg (5-10 mg) IV over 2 min (if no effect after 15 min)
    - Max: 30 mg IV total; Onset: 1-5 min; Duration: 10 – 20 min

- – Diltiazem
  - Initial dose: 10 mg to 20 mg IV bolus (0.25 mg/kg dose over 2 min)
  - 2nd dose: 15 mg to 25 mg IV push (0.35 mg/kg) 15 min later PRN
  - Infusion: 5 mg/hr, titrate by 5 mg/hr q15 min, safe in lower blood pressures
  - Max: 15 mg/hr; Onset: 3 min; Duration: 1-3 hrs (bolus); 1-10 hrs (after continuous infusion, prolonged if infusion >24 hrs)
- β-blockers can be used as first- or second-line treatment. Use caution in asthmatics.
  - – Metoprolol
    - Initial dose: 5 mg IV, may repeat q10 min, max 20 mg
    - Start oral regimen of 50-100 mg after successful conversion of SVT.
  - – Esmolol
    - Loading dose: 500 mcg/kg IV bolus over 1 min (can repeat loading dose once)
    - Infusion: 50 mcg/kg/min, titrate by 50 mcg/kg/min q4 min
    - Max: 300 mcg/kg/min; Onset: 1-2 min; Duration: 10-30 min

Second-line recommendations
- Procainamide (preferred over calcium channel blockers and β-blockers in wide QRS SVT)
  - – Loading dose:
    - 100 mg IV over 2 min q5 min **OR** 20-50 mg/min for 20-35 min
    - Give dose(s) until arrhythmia is controlled, QRS interval widens 50%, arrhythmia is suppressed, prolonged QT interval, hypotension, or max dose (17 mg/kg or 1000 mg).
    - Reduce loading dose to 12 mg/kg in patients with renal impairment.
  - – Infusion: 1-4 mg/min
    - Avoid in patients with prolonged QT interval and/or congestive heart failure.
- Flecanide: 2 mg/kg over a 10-min period
- Propafenone: 2 mg/kg over a 10-min period
  - – Amiodarone: 150 mg over a 10-min period followed by 1 mg/min for 6 hours, **THEN** 0.5 mg/min for 18 hours

SVT+AV Node Re-entry/Pre-excitation
- Procainamide (preferred over CCB and β-blockers in wide QRS SVT)
  - – Loading dose:
    - 100 mg IV over 2 min q5 min **OR** 20-50 mg/min for 20-35 min
    - Give dose(s) until arrhythmia is controlled, QRS interval widens 50%, arrhythmia suppressed, prolonged QT interval, hypotension, or max dose (17 mg/kg or 1000 mg).
    - Reduce loading dose to 12 mg/kg in patients with renal impairment.
  - – Infusion: 1-4 mg/min
  - – Max: 1 g load or 9 g/day maintenance

→ SVT can produce diffuse ST depression with ST elevation in aVR mimicking ischemia, which is completely rate-related. ECG should normalize after successful cardioversion; biomarkers should not be analyzed if ECG normalized.

→ Calcium channel and beta blockers should be used with caution in CHF patients (may worsen heart failure).

→ Identify the precipitant of SVT based on the patient's presentation. Consider structural heart disease, pulmonary embolism, thyroid disease, pregnancy, medications, alcohol withdrawal, and sepsis as possible causes.

→ All medications listed — except amiodarone — are pregnancy category C and considered safe for use.

→ Avoid combination of AV nodal blocking agent with long duration of action (i.e., calcium channel blockers and β-blockers), as profound bradycardia may develop.

VENTRICULAR TACHYCARDIA (VT)
Cardiogenic Shock

Unstable ventricular dysrhythmias
• VT is defined as a patient with tachycardia-induced hypotension, altered mental status, acute CHF, ischemic chest pain, or myocardial ischemia.
• Consider sedation prior to cardioversion.
  – Midazolam: 2-4 mg IV bolus
  – Etomidate: 0.15 mg/kg IV x 1
  – Propofol: 0.5-1 mg/kg IV x 1 (caution with hypotensive patient)
• Perform synchronized cardioversion at 360J with monophasic defibrillator (or biphasic equivalent).
• If patient pulseless, perform ACLS for ventricular fibrillation (VF)/pulseless VT.

Stable ventricular dysrhythmias
Sustained monomorphic ventricular tachycardia
• Procainamide: Class IA – Na+ channel blocker, recommended in AVNRT and undifferentiated wide-complex tachycardia
  – Loading dose:
    ▪ 100 mg/dose IV over 2 min q5 min; *OR* 20-50 mg/min for 25-30 min (max infusion rate 50 mg/min)
    ▪ Give dose(s) until dysrhythmia is controlled, QRS interval widens 50%, dysrhythmia is suppressed, QT interval prolongs, hypotension, or max dose (17 mg/kg or 1000 mg).
    ▪ Reduce loading dose to 12 mg/kg in patients with renal impairment.
  – Infusion: 1-4 mg/min
  – Max: 1 g load *OR* 9 g/day maintenance
    ▪ Avoid in patients with prolonged QT interval and/or congestive heart failure.

- Amiodarone (Class III)
  - Loading dose: 150 mg IV over 10 min
  - Infusion: 1 mg/min IV over 6 hrs, *THEN* 0.5 mg/min x 18 hrs
  - Max: 2.2 g over 24 hrs
- Lidocaine (Class IB; Na+ channel blocker; second-line agent)
  - Loading dose: 1-1.5 mg/kg IV over 2-3 minutes, repeat 0.5-0.75 mg/kg IV every 5-10 min; max cumulative dose: 3 mg/kg
  - Infusion: 1-4 mg/min IV
  - Max: 300 mg total dose in 1 hr

Additional therapeutic options and considerations
- Adenosine
  - Initial dose: 6 mg IV push over 1-3 sec; may repeat at 12 mg IV every 1-2 min if no conversion
    - Avoid giving for unstable or irregular/polymorphic wide-complex tachycardias, as it may cause ventricular fibrillation.
    - Keep defibrillator in close proximity.

Polymorphic ventricular tachycardia
- *Polymorphic VT associated with prolonged QT interval (>600 ms)*
  - Magnesium sulfate
    - Initial dose: 1-2 g IV over 15 min
    - Assess for factors that prolong the QT interval (e.g., medications, hypokalemia, hypomagnesemia)
- *Polymorphic VT associated with normal QT interval*
  - Amiodarone
    - Loading dose: 150 mg IV x 1 over 10 min
    - Infusion: 1 mg/min IV x 6 hrs, *THEN* 0.5 mg/min x 18 hrs
      - May repeat 150 mg IV if tachyarrhythmia recurs.
    - Max: 2.2 g over 24 hrs

PEARLS
→ Replete electrolyte deficiencies (esp. potassium and magnesium) in patients with ventricular dysrhythmias.
→ Avoid calcium channel blockers (e.g., verapamil, diltiazem) and AV nodal blocking drugs (e.g., digoxin, adenosine) for wide-complex tachycardias of unknown origin (N.B. Consider WPW and AVNRT as potential etiologies).
→ Treat wide-complex tachycardias as VT if the diagnosis is unclear.
→ A magnet placed over an ICD/pacemaker disables "sensing" and may terminate VT secondary to oversensing of atrial rhythms.
→ Avoid placing pads over ICDs → use anterior-posterior placement.

ACUTE ISCHEMIC STROKE

Treatment

- *Thrombolysis*
  - Recombinant tissue-type plasminogen activator (rt-PA, alteplase)
    - Total dose: 0.9 mg/kg IV (actual body weight), max 90 mg
      - Bolus: 10% of dose (0.09 mg/kg up to 9 mg) IV over 1 min
      - Infusion: remaining dose (0.81 mg/kg up to 81 mg) IV over 60 min
      - Review contraindications below *(Table 2)*.

Table 2: Contraindications for t-PA in Acute Ischemic CVA
Exclusion criteria
• Head trauma or prior stroke in previous 3 months
• Patient has a known history of intracranial hemorrhage
• Patient has symptoms suggestive of subarachnoid hemorrhage
• Patient had a seizure at the onset of stroke
• Arterial puncture at non-compressible site in previous 7 days
• SBP >185 mmHg or DBP >110 mmHg
• Evidence of active bleeding
• Acute bleeding diathesis: platelets <100,000, active anticoagulant use with INR>1.7 or PT >15 sec, heparin use within 48 hrs with aPTT >ULN
• Glucose <50 mg/dL of >400 mg/dL
• CT with multi-lobar infarction >1/3 cerebral hemisphere
Relative exclusion criteria
• Minor or rapidly improving stroke symptoms
• Patient has a large stroke with NIH Stroke Scale score >22
• Recent acute MI within 3 months
• Major surgery, serious trauma <14 days
• Recent GI or GU hemorrhage <21 days

- *Blood pressure management*
  - Nicardipine
    - Infusion: 5 mg/hr, titrate by 2.5 mg/hr q5-15 min
    - Max: 15 mg/hr; Onset: 1-2 min; Duration: 40 min
  - Labetalol
    - Loading dose: 20 mg IV, double dose at 10-min intervals to max of 300 mg
    - Infusion: 2-8 mg/min, titrate by 0.5 mg/min q10 min
    - Max: 8 mg/min; Onset: 2-5 min; Duration 2-4 hrs
      - *Note: Consider alternative agents if patient remains on a high dose of labetalol.*

- Esmolol
  - Loading dose: 250-500 mcg/kg IV over 1 min
  - Infusion: 50 mcg/kg/min, titrate by *repeating loading dose* (for rapid response) q4 min and increase infusion by 50 mcg/kg/min
    - Skip repeat loading doses as BP approaches goal.
  - Max: 300 mcg/kg/min
- Enalaprilat
  - Initial dose: 1.25 mg IV over 5 min, titrated up to 5 mg/dose q6 hrs
    - If receiving diuretic: 0.625 mg IV over 5 min, repeat dose if inadequate in 1 hr and increase to 1.25 mg IV q6 hrs.

Additional therapeutics and considerations

- Consider IV rt-PA if symptom onset is within 3-4.5 hrs and age <80 years.
- For patients receiving thrombolysis: SBP goal <180 mmHg, DBP goal <105 mmHg. For patients not receiving thrombolysis: SBP goal ≤220 mmHg, DBP goal ≤120 mmHg, but avoid lowering BP by more than 15-25% within the first 24 hrs after stroke onset.
- Avoid use of nitroprusside and nitroglycerin due to the possibility of increasing intracranial pressure through venodilation.
- Patients receiving IV thrombolysis should have frequent neurologic examinations to monitor for hemorrhagic transformation. Avoid anticoagulants and antiplatelet medications within 24 hrs of rt-PA.
- Use insulin for glycemic control if serum glucose >185 mg/dL; avoid hypoglycemia.

PEARLS

→ IV rt-PA benefit is time-dependent; door-to-needle time of bolus administration goal is within 60 minutes.

→ Consider obtaining multimodal CT or MRI to improve diagnostic accuracy; however, do not delay emergent treatment to obtain imaging studies.

→ Weigh the patient as soon as possible and prepare the rt-PA doses prior to imaging in order to decrease time to drug; the manufacturer has agreed to replace doses that are not used.

→ Consider intra-arterial thrombolysis for selected patients with major stroke of <6 hrs duration who are not otherwise candidates for intravenous rt-PA.

→ Patients receiving novel oral anticoagulants (dabigatran, rivaroxaban, apixaban) may have normal or only minimally elevated INR, aPTT/PT in the setting of therapeutic anticoagulation. The risks and benefits of intravenous thrombolysis in these patients must be considered carefully on a case-by-case basis.

→ Nicardipine efficacy may be compromised with concurrent hepatic-enzyme-inducing drugs (phenytoin, carbamazepine).

→ Up to 5% of patients on ACE inhibitors may be at increased risk for orolingual angioedema with concurrent rt-P.

ANEURYSMAL SUBARACHNOID HEMORRHAGE

Treatment

Blood pressure management: Goal SBP <160 mmHg, MAP <110 mmHg

- Nicardipine
  - Infusion: 5 mg/hr, titrate by 2.5 mg/hr q5-15 min
  - Max: 15 mg/hr; Onset: 1-2 min; Duration: 40 min
- Labetalol
  - Loading dose: 20 mg IV, double dose at 10-min intervals to max of 300 mg
  - Infusion: 2-8 mg/min, titrate by 0.5 mg/min q10 min
  - Max: 8 mg/min; Onset: 2-5 min; Duration: 2-4 hrs
    - *Note: Consider alternative agents if patient remains on a high dose of labetalol.*
- Esmolol
  - Loading dose: 250-500 mcg/kg IV over 1 min
  - Infusion: 50 mcg/kg/min, titrate by *repeating loading dose* (for rapid response) q4 min and increase infusion by 50 mcg/kg/min
    - Skip repeat loading doses as BP approaches goal.
  - Max: 300 mcg/kg/min
- Enalaprilat
  - Initial dose: 1.25 mg IV over 5 min, titrated up to 5 mg/dose q6 hrs
    - If receiving diuretic: 0.625 mg IV over 5 min, repeat dose if inadequate in 1 hr and increase to 1.25 mg IV q6 hrs.

Increased intracranial pressure, signs of herniation

- Mannitol (20%)
  - Initial dose: 1 g/kg IV bolus
  - May repeat 0.5-1 g/kg IV as needed q6-8 hrs for increased ICP so long as serum Osm <320.
  - Replace urinary losses with isotonic fluids to avoid intravascular volume depletion and hypotension.
- Hypertonic saline (3%): 250 mL infused over 20-30 min

Seizures: For clinical or suspected seizures

- Levetiracetam
  - Loading dose: 20 mg/kg IV (round to nearest 250 mg) over 60 min
  - Repeat dosing: 500-1000 mg IV/PO q12 hrs
- Phenytoin (IV/PO)/fosphenytoin (in PE, IV only)
  - Loading dose: 20 mg/kg IV at max rate of 50 mg/min (phenytoin) or over 60 min (fosphenytoin). Repeat dosing: 5 mg/kg/day in 3 divided doses (100 mg IV/PO q8 hrs)
  - Obtain level 1 hour after loading dose (therapeutic range: 10-20 mcg/mL). Consider monitoring free levels with end-organ dysfunction or low albumin.

Delayed cerebral ischemia prevention

- Nimodipine
  - Dose: 60 mg PO/enteral tube q4 hr x 21 days
    - May be given 30 mg PO/enteral q2 hr if BP does not tolerate 60 mg dose.
    - Has been FATAL when given IV.

Additional therapeutic options and considerations

- Surgical clipping or endovascular coiling of the ruptured aneurysm should be performed as early as feasible to reduce the rate of re-bleeding. If there will be a considerable delay, use of tranexamic acid or aminocaproic acid may be considered after discussion with neurosurgical consultant.
- CSF diversion with ventriculostomy is recommended for acute hydrocephalus. Consider this early in patients who have intraventricular blood present on CT scan.
- Maintain euvolemia with isotonic fluids to prevent cerebral vasospasm and delayed cerebral ischemia.
- For hyponatremia: Limit free water intake while maintaining euvolemia. Hypertonic saline IV may be used. Avoid correcting serum sodium more than 12-24 mmol/L in 24 hrs to avoid central pontine myelinolysis.
- Use insulin for glycemic control if serum glucose >185 mg/dL; avoid hypoglycemia.

PEARLS

→ Risk of re-bleeding is highest in the first 24 hours after the initial hemorrhage.

→ Morbidity and mortality are associated with re-bleeding, increased intracranial pressure, vasospasm and delayed cerebral ischemia, seizures, hyponatremia, cardiac abnormalities, hyperthermia, hypothalamic dysfunction, and pituitary insufficiency.

→ BP should be controlled with a titratable agent to balance the risk of stroke, hypertension-related bleeding, and to maintain cerebral perfusion pressure.

→ Avoid the use of nitroprusside and nitroglycerin due to the possibility of increasing intracranial pressure through venodilation.

→ Beware of SAH-associated myocardial stunning, which can lead to neurogenic pulmonary edema. Perform bedside echocardiogram if clinically suspected.

CEREBRAL EDEMA (INCREASED ICP/HERNIATION)

Treatment

Blood pressure management
- Maintain systolic blood pressure (SBP) between 140 and 160 mmHg and cerebral perfusion pressure (CPP) >70.
- Nicardipine
  - Infusion: 5 mg/hr, titrate by 2.5 mg/hr q10-15 min
  - Max: 15 mg/hr; Onset: 1-2 min; Duration: 40 min
- Labetalol
  - Loading dose: 20 mg IV, double dose q10 min to max of 300 mg
  - Infusion: 2-8 mg/min, titrate by 0.5 mg/min q10 min
  - Max: 8 mg/min; Onset: 2-5 min; Duration 2-4 hrs
    - Note: Consider alternative agents if patient remains on a high dose of labetalol.

Osmotherapy
- Hypertonic saline: target serum Na of 145-155 mEq/L with persistent symptoms of cerebral edema
  - 23.4% NaCl: 30 mL IV bolus over 20-30 min, Max: 2 doses
  - 3% NaCl: 3 mL/kg IV bolus over 20 min
  - 7.5% NaCl: 1 mL/kg IV bolus over 20 min
- Mannitol (20%)
  - Loading dose: 0.25-1 g/kg bolus
  - Repeat bolus 0.25-0.5 g/kg IV q4-6 hrs
    - Upper limit serum osmolality: 315-320 mOsm

Additional therapeutic options and considerations
- Raise the head of bed to 30 degrees and prevent hyperthermia (>38°C).
- Consider short-term mild hyperventilation to maintain $PaCO_2$ 30-35 mmHg.
- Seizure prophylaxis with the following:
  - Levetiracetam: 20 mg/kg IV loading dose over 60 min
  - Phenytoin: 20 mg/kg IV loading dose at max rate of 50 mg/min
  - Fosphenytoin: 20 mg/kg PE IV loading dose over 60 min
- For refractory symptoms consider: hypothermia (33°C-36°C), paralytics, barbiturate coma with pentobarbital (10 mg/kg IV loading dose slowly over 30 mins **OR** ≤25 mg/min, **THEN** 5 mg/kg every hour x3 doses, **THEN** maintenance 1-4 mg/kg/hr); continuous EEG monitoring for patients with abnormal mental status.

PEARLS

→ Disadvantage of hypertonic saline: need central line for infusion of 7.5% or greater concentrations due to risk of phlebitis and tissue necrosis. Some institutions allow 3% via peripheral IV, but typically at slower rates than recommended for this indication.

→ Disadvantage of mannitol: volume contraction from osmotic diuresis, risk of renal failure, theoretical rebound cerebral edema.

→ Current evidence shows that hypertonic saline may be more effective than mannitol in the treatment of intracranial hypertension, and should be considered in multi-trauma or TBI patients in the setting of hypovolemia.

STATUS EPILEPTICUS

Indications
- Persistent seizure: >5 min
- Recurrent seizures: without return to consciousness within 5 min

Treatment
- Lorazepam: 4 mg IV bolus slowly over 2 min; may repeat in 10-15 min
  - Preferred because of longer duration of anticonvulsant effect.
- Diazepam: 5-10 mg IV; may repeat in 5-10 min
- Midazolam: 10 mg deep IM into large muscle if no IV access can be obtained
  - Can also be administered via intranasal or buccal routes.

AND simultaneous
- Fosphenytoin: 20 mg/kg PE (phenytoin equivalents) IV at a rate of 150 mg/min PE
  OR
- Phenytoin: 20 mg/kg IV at max rate of 50 mg/min; slower if hypotension, cardiac arrhythmias
  - If seizure lasts >10 min, an additional dose of 10 mg/kg PE of fosphenytoin or phenytoin can be given.
- Valproic acid (valproate sodium)
  - Loading dose: 20-30 mg/kg IV at a rate of 40 mg/min
  - Consider for patients who are on chronic valproate therapy.

Refractory status epilepticus (SE)
- *If the patient does not respond to optimal benzodiazepine and phenytoin (or fosphenytoin) loading after 20 min, intubation is required and EEG monitoring is recommended.*
- Midazolam
  - Loading dose: 0.2 mg/kg IV bolus (at a rate of 2 mg/min)
  - Maintenance infusion: 0.05-0.6 mg/kg/hr IV to goal of seizure cessation
- Propofol
  - Loading dose: 1-2 mg/kg IV over 5 min
  - Infusion: begin at 20 mcg/kg/min; may titrate by 5-10 mcg/kg/min every 5 min to goal of seizure cessation (max 200 mcg/kg/min)
  - Caution in doses >80 mcg/kg/min for >48 hours
- Phenobarbital
  - Initial dose: 20 mg/kg IV at max rate of ≤60 mg/min (slower in elderly, <60 kg)
  - May given an additional dose of 5-10 mg/kg if seizures persist >10 min. Monitor for hypotension, sedation, and hypoventilation.
- Phenobarbital
  - Initial dose: 5-15 mg/kg at a rate of ≤50 mg/min; may give an additional 5-10 mg/kg
  - Maintenance infusion: 0.5-5 mg/kg/hr
  - Anticipate hypotension requiring vasopressor support.

Additional therapeutic options and considerations
- Levetiracetam: 1000-3000 mg IV at a rate of 2-5 mg/kg/min

PEARLS

→ Nonconvulsive SE (NSE) should be strongly considered if exam does not correlate with the clinical situation within 20-30 min after seizure cessation.

→ Toxins associated with SE include: bupropion, monoamine oxidase inhibitors, isoniazid (INH), and theophylline (all classically do not respond to phenytoin or fosphenytoin).

→ Treat INH-induced SE with pyridoxine (vitamin B6) at an empiric dose of 5 g slow IV at 0.5-1 g/min in concert with diazepam. Contact the Poison Control Center.

→ For alcohol-withdrawal seizures, use phenobarbital as second-line therapy.

→ Seizures may be a sign of eclampsia after 20 weeks' gestation. Load with 4-6 g magnesium sulfate IV over 15-20 min (over 3-4 min if eclampsia is severe) followed by infusion of 1-2 g/hr.

→ Loading does do not require adjustment for hepatic or renal insufficiency.

→ Avoid paralytics (except short-acting for RSI).

→ Perform blood glucose testing at presentation.

TRAUMATIC SPINAL CORD INJURY (SCI)

Indications
- Spinal shock: loss of neurological function below level of SCI; transient process that can last from days to months
- Neurogenic shock: hemodynamic instability and autonomic dysfunction that is associated with SCI
- Clinical triad of:
  - Hypotension
  - Relative bradycardia
  - Hypothermia
- Prevention of secondary injury

Treatment
- ***Airway/breathing:*** Maintain airway patency and oxygenation.
- ***Blood pressure management:*** Maintain MAP ≥90 mmHg to prevent cord ischemia.
  - Fluid resuscitation: 0.9% NaCl (normal saline) IV
    - Excessive fluid can worsen cord edema.
  - Vasopressors if not responsive to fluid:
    - Dopamine: β >α at low dose, *use when bradycardic*
      - Infusion: 5-10 mcg/kg/min IV, titrate by 5 mcg/kg/min q10 min
      - Max dose: 50 mcg/kg/min; Onset: <5 min; Duration: <10 min
    - Norepinephrine: α >β
      - Infusion: 0.05 mcg/kg/min IV, titrate by 0.02 mcg/kg/min q5 min
      - Dose range: 0.05-0.5 mcg/kg/min; Onset: 1-2 min; Duration: 1-2 min

- No true max, but consider using additional agents if patient is unresponsive to higher doses.
  - Phenylephrine: α only
    - Infusion: 100-180 mcg/min, titrate by 25 mcg/min q10 min
    - Weight-based dosing: 0.5 mcg/kg/min, titrate to response
    - Dose range: 0.5-9 mcg/kg/min; Onset: 1-2 min; Duration: 15-20 min
    - Adverse effect: reflex bradycardia
  - Epinephrine: β1>β2 and α, *for refractory hypotension*
    - Infusion: 0.05 mcg/kg/min IV, titrate by 0.02-0.05 mcg/kg/min q15 min
    - Dose range: 0.05-0.5 mcg/kg/min; Onset: 1-2 min; Duration: 5-10 min
    - No true max, but consider using additional agents if patient is unresponsive to higher doses.
  - Vasopressin: 0.04 units/min; for refractory hypotension; do not titrate
- *Heart rate control: Prevent bradycardia*
  - Atropine: 0.5-1 mg rapid IV bolus q3-5 min, up to max 0.04 mg/kg (or 3 mg)
  - Consider transvenous pacing if patient is refractory to pharmacologic treatment.

Additional therapeutic options and considerations

- Methylprednisolone
  - Indication: non-penetrating trauma within 8 hrs of injury
  - Contraindications: penetrating trauma, moderate to severe traumatic brain injury, and other comorbidities associated with complications from glucocorticoid administration
  - Initial dose: 30 mg/kg IV bolus over 15 min
  - Infusion: 5.4 mg/kg/hr IV for 23 hrs starting 45 min after bolus
    - *Controversial:* Discuss with consultants before administering; consider local protocols.
    - Increases risk of complications with uncertain neurological benefits, thus no longer recommended by many society guidelines.
- Avoid complications: Place Foley catheter and nasogastric tube as needed; prophylaxis for peptic ulcer, deep vein thrombosis (with low molecular weight heparin), and constipation; precautions for ventilator-associated pneumonia.

PEARLS

→ *Neurogenic* spinal shock is a diagnosis of exclusion.
→ Rule out hemorrhage and other causes of shock (tamponade, pneumothorax, etc.).
→ If injury is below T6, then hypotension is not likely from spinal shock.
→ Injuries above T6 warrant vasopressors with both inotropic and vasoconstrictive properties.
→ Monitor for delayed respiratory failure secondary to ascending cord edema.
→ Document: motor exam, sensation, reflexes, perianal sensation, rectal tone, and anogenital reflex.

DIABETIC KETOACIDOSIS

Treatment

- *Fluid resuscitation*
  - 0.9% Normal saline (NS) IV bolus (start by administering 2 L and target a MAP of >65; typically 6-8 L needed to replace fluid deficit)
    - Once MAP goal achieved, continue NS (½ NS if patient is hypernatremic) at 150-300 mL/hr and titrate to urine output of 1-2 ml/kg/hr.
    - Transition to D_5 ½ NS at 100-200 mL/hr once serum glucose approaches 200-250 mg/dL.
- *Hyperglycemia/anion gap*
  - Regular insulin
    - Continuous infusion: 0.1-0.14 unit/kg/hr IV (0.3 units/kg IM), no bolus necessary as initial insulin bolus has not been demonstrated to be advantageous versus no insulin bolus.
      - Target glucose reduction rate of 100-200 mg/dL/hr, monitor q1 hr finger sticks
      - If glucose falls <50 mg/dL/hr then double insulin dose.
      - Increase 2-3x if no response by 2-4 hrs.
      - Once glucose is approximately 200-250 mg/dL, decrease insulin to 0.05-0.1 units/kg/hr to maintain glucose between 150 and 200 mg/dL.
      - May need to hold insulin if glucose is <150 mg/dL.
  - Long-acting insulin
    - Administer long-acting insulin glargine (1 unit/kg/day SQ) after evidence of DKA resolution (see below).
- *Electrolyte management* (monitor q2 hrs)
  - Potassium
    - K >5.3 mEq/L: no KCl/K-Phos, recheck q2 hrs
    - K 3.3-5.3 mEq/L: start KCl/K-Phos @ 20-30 mEq/L/hr (can be added to IV fluids)
    - K <3.3 mEq/L: start KCl/K-Phos @ 20-30 mEq/L/hr and hold insulin until K >3.3 mEq/L
    - Cautiously replace electrolytes in patients with renal insufficiency.
  - Phosphorus
    - Replace if <1.0 mg/dL: add 20-30 mEq/L to IVF.
    - Replacement can precipitate hypocalcemia: monitor serum Ca^{2+} levels.
  - Sodium bicarbonate – *controversial*
    - If pH >7.0: no $NaHCO_3$
    - If pH is 6.9-7.0: consider 75 mEq (1.5 amp) $NaHCO_3$ with 10 mEq K in 1000 mL of sterile water.
      - Administer over 1 hour until pH >7.0.

- If pH <6.9: consider 100 mEq (2 amps) NaHCO₃ with 20 mEq K in 400 mL of sterile water given.
  - Administer at 200 mL/hr until pH >7.0.
- **Evidence of DKA resolution**
  - Blood glucose <200 mg/dL plus **TWO** of the following:
    - Arterial pH >7.3
    - Serum bicarbonate >15 mEq/L
    - Anion gap <12 mEq/L

Additional therapeutic options and considerations

- Rapid fluid correction may cause cerebral edema. Look for these warning signs: severe headache, vomiting, hypertension, or change in mental status.
  - Dx: CT/MRI
  - Treatment: mannitol 1 gm/kg IV bolus
- Please refer to the ISPAD Protocol for the treatment of pediatric DKA.

PEARLS

→ Pseudohyponatremia correction formula: for every 100 the glucose is over 100, **ADD** 1.6 to the serum Na value.

→ Acetoacetate is the ketone that is measured; however, the first ketone produced is β-hydroxybutyrate (β-HOB). β-HOB is converted to acetoacetate. As a result, the anion gap decreases (ketones are metabolized) as the measured ketones increase (β-HOB is being converted to acetoacetate).

→ Insulin bolus has *not* been shown to be beneficial in clinical management.

→ DKA is often precipitated by pregnancy, infection, myocardial infarction, dietary changes, or medication non-compliance. Search for an underlying cause while concurrently treating the DKA.

HYPERNATREMIA

Treatment

- **Volume-depleted** (most common)
  - Treat hypotensive patients with 0.9% normal saline bolus of 1-2 liters.
  - When hemodynamically stable, calculate free-water deficit and use hypotonic IV fluid D5W or ½ NS to replace half of the free-water deficit over the first 24 hours and the remaining half over the subsequent 24 hrs.
    - Free-water deficit (L) = TBW (total body water) x (plasma Na/140-1)
      - Male TBW (L) = 0.6 x body weight (kg)
      - Female or elderly: TBW (L) = 0.5 x body weight (kg)
  - Supplement with PO/NG/OG free water in patients who are not altered.
- **Euvolemic/secondary to central diabetes insipidus (DI)**
  - Desmopressin (DDAVP) – first line
    - Chronic therapy
      - Intravenous: 0.1-1 mcg bid
      - Intranasal: 10-20 mcg QD or bid
      - Subcutaneous: 1-2 mcg bid
      - Oral: 0.05 mg bid (0.1-1.5 mg bid-tid)
  - Vasopressin
    - IM/subcutaneous: Starting dose 5-10 units 2-4 times/day as needed
    - Titrate based on UOP: goal daily UOP <3.0 L
  - Salt restriction: <2.3 g sodium/day
- **Hypovolemic** (iatrogenic secondary to large sodium or bicarbonate gains)
  - Promote sodium removal
    - Bolus-dose furosemide: 40 mg IV dose **OR** 2x patient's home oral dose
    - Continuous infusion:
      - Initial dose: 40 mg IV bolus, titrate by 5-20 mg/hr
      - Goal: UOP >0.5 mL/kg/hr, follow electrolytes closely
  - Supplement free water (D5W) to prevent excessive water loss from diuresis.
  - Some patients may require hemodialysis if in renal failure

Additional therapeutic options and considerations

- Rapid correction of sodium may cause cerebral edema; maximum rate of correction should be no more than 2 mEq/L per hr.
- Reverse chronic (or unknown duration) hyponatremia at 0.5 mEq/L per hr to a total of 10-12 mEq/day.
- Nephrogenic DI may require dialysis.

PEARLS

→ Diabetic patients may need insulin along with D5W infusion to prevent osmotic diuresis.
→ Hypernatremia <24 hours should be corrected in 24 hours. If >24 hours or unknown duration, correct over 48 hours.
→ Normal saline should be used in hypotensive patients only; once hemodynamically stable, change to a hypotonic fluid.
→ Central DI responds to exogenous ADH, whereas nephrogenic DI does not.

HYPONATREMIA

Initial Approach (Na <135 mEq/L)

- Check serum osmolality (OSM).
  - If OSM normal or high (i.e., isotonic or hypertonic hyponatremia), consider elevated proteins, lipids, glucose, or lab error.
  - If OSM low (hypotonic hyponatremia), consider volume status to distinguish:
    - Hypovolemic (e.g., vomiting, diarrhea, diuretics)
    - Euvolemic (SIADH)
    - Hypervolemic (e.g., CHF, cirrhosis, renal failure)
- Check labs: BMP, TSH, cortisol, uric acid (if diuretics)
- Check urine: UA, electrolytes, urea, creatinine, osmolality, uric acid (if diuretics)
- Differentiate symptomatic vs. asymptomatic
- **Max Na correction 0.5 mEq/L/hr (12 mEq/L *total*) in first 24 hrs**

Treatment

- Severe symptoms (AMS, seizures, neurologic deficits)
  - Hypertonic saline (3%)
    - 100 mL over 10 min IV; repeat up to 2x until symptoms resolve
    - ***THEN*** 100 mL over 1 hr
    - *Each 100 mL will raise Na ~2 mEq/L*
- Mild/moderate symptoms (lethargy, dizziness)
  - 0.9% NaCl 500-1,000 mL/h (if hypovolemic)
    - Once euvolemic, ADH will be suppressed, which may further elevate Na.
  - *Consider 3% NaCl IV*
    - 1-2 mL/kg/h (max correction 6-12 mEq/L in first 24 hrs)
    - Recheck Na levels every 1-2 hrs (watch closely).
- Asymptomatic
  - Hypotonic, hypovolemic: Administer 0.9% NaCl 500-1,000 mL/h until euvolemic
    - Recheck Na levels every 1-2 hrs.
  - Hypotonic, euvolemic: Free H_2O restriction (<800 mL/day), +/- vasopressin
  - Hypotonic, hypervolemic: Free H_2O restriction (<800 mL/day), +/- mild diuresis
  - Isotonic/hypertonic: Treat underlying cause (see above).

Additional considerations

- Most accurate way to determine how much Na to give:
  - Change in serum Na (with 1 L of infusate) = (infusate Na – serum Na) / (TBW + 1)
    - Male TBW (L) = 0.6 x body weight (kg)
    - Female (or elderly) TBW (L) = 0.5 x body weight (kg)
    - Infusate Na: 3% NaCl (513), 0.9% NaCl (154)
- Urine Na <20 suggests a non-renal etiology.
- Urine Na >20 suggests a renal etiology (though >40 may be SIADH).

→ Rule of 6s:
  – 6-a-day makes sense for safety (goal max Na increase of 6 mEq/L in 24 hrs)
  – 6 in 6 hours for severe symptoms and stop (max Na increase of 6 mEq/L in 6 hrs)
→ If in doubt and patient is asymptomatic, then just restrict free H_2O.

NEUROLEPTIC MALIGNANT SYNDROME

Indication

Idiosyncratic reaction with use of dopamine antagonists (e.g., antipsychotics) *OR* discontinuation of dopamine agonists (e.g., levodopa/carbidopa). Various diagnostic criteria have been proposed and presentations are variable, but the majority of patients present with the following tetrad over 1-3 days:

• Fever (most common feature)
• "Lead-pipe" muscle rigidity (less commonly dyskinesia, akinesia, etc. are present)
• Altered mental status
• Autonomic dysfunction

Treatment

• Discontinuation of dopaminergic antagonist *OR* reinstitution of dopamine agonist
• Supportive care with aggressive cooling and adequate volume resuscitation for likely rhabdomyolysis
• Benzodiazepines (first line: attenuates sympathetic hyperactivity)
  – Lorazepam: 2-4 mg IV push q10-15 min, max: 12 mg
  – Diazepam: 0.2 mg/kg IV (5-10 mg IV, repeat in 3-4 hrs), max: 10 mg
• Dantrolene (↓ skeletal muscle activity by inhibiting ryanodine receptor calcium channels)
  – Initial dose: 1-2.5 mg/kg IV q6 hrs x 48 hrs (maximum dose: 10 mg/kg/day)
  – Maintenance dose: 1 mg/kg (4-8 mg/kg/day in 4 doses x 1-3 days) PO q6 hrs
    ▪ Use with caution in patients taking calcium-channel blockers.
    ▪ Hepatotoxicity can occur at high dosages.
• Bromocriptine (centrally acting dopamine agonist)
  – Initial dose: 2.5-10 mg PO q8 hrs; Max: 45 mg/day
• Amantadine: 200 mg PO q12 hrs
  – Postulated to block dopamine reuptake or increase dopamine release

→ Avoid succinylcholine for intubation given theoretical (although unlikely) relationship to malignant hyperthermia and potentiation of rhabdomyolysis.
→ Common findings include elevated WBC, ALT, AST, CK, renal failure, seizures and rhabdomyolysis.

→ Serotonin syndrome is classically associated with a rapid onset, hyperreflexia, myoclonus, shivering, and without elevated CK.

→ Consider electroconvulsive therapy (reports of resolution with three or four sessions, but efficacy and indications are speculative), **OR** levodopa + amantadine (dopaminergic agonists).

→ Common drugs associated with NMS:
  - Neuroleptics/antipsychotics (e.g., haldol, fluphenazine)
  - Typical antipsychotics (e.g., chlorpromazine, loxapine)
  - Atypical antipsychotics (e.g., aripiprazole, olanazapine, quetiapine, risperidone)
  - Dopamine antagonists (e.g., metoclopramide, prochlorperazine, promethazine)

MESENTERIC ISCHEMIA
Distributive/Septic shock (if bowel necrosis is present)

Treatment
General management for mesenteric ischemia of any etiology
- Aggressive fluid resuscitation: 0.9% normal saline IV bolus
- Broad-spectrum antibiotics that have coverage for bowel flora should be used and instituted early.
    - Piperacillin/tazobactam: 3.375 mg IV q6 hrs **OR**
    - Cefepime: 2 g IV q8 hrs **PLUS** metronidazole: 500 mg IV q6 hrs
- NGT placement for decompression
- Blood pressure management (goal MAP >65 mmHg)
    - Vasopressor therapy: avoid using vasopressin and α-agonists.
        - Norepinephrine:
            - Infusion: 0.05 mcg/kg/min IV, titrate by 0.02 mcg/kg/min q5 min
            - Max: none, but avoid high doses; Onset: 1-2 min; Duration: 1-2 min

Acute arterial mesenteric ischemia
- Heparin (unfractionated):
    - Loading dose: 80 units/kg IV bolus
    - Infusion: initiate at 18 units/kg/hr IV (goal aPTT 2-3x normal)
- Additional therapeutic options and considerations:
    - Glucagon: may help reduce the associated vasospasm
        - Infusion: 1 mcg/kg/min IV
        - Max: 10 mcg/kg/min
    - *In conjunction with angiography through a selective intra-arterial (IA) catheter at the site of occlusion*
        - Papaverine: PDE-inhibitor causing smooth-muscle dilation
            - Infusion: 30-60 mg/hr intra-arterial transcatheter delivery
        - Alteplase (rt-PA):
            - Loading dose: 2-5 mg IA transcatheter delivery
            - Infusion: 1-2 mg/hr by IA transcatheter delivery

Non-occlusive mesenteric ischemia
- Address predisposing factors:
    - Correct hypoperfusion (sepsis, heart failure, hypovolemia).
    - Discontinue offending medications (α-blockers and other vasopressors, digitalis, and ergotamine).
    - *Use in conjunction with angiography through a selective intra-arterial (IA) catheter at the site of occlusion.*
        - Papaverine: PDE-inhibitor causing smooth-muscle dilation
            - Infusion: 30-60 mg/hr intra-arterial transcatheter delivery

Mesenteric venous thrombosis
- Heparin (unfractionated):
  - Loading dose: 80 units/kg IV bolus
  - Infusion: 18 units/kg/hr IV (goal aPTT 2-3x normal)
- In conjunction with angiography through a selective intra-arterial (IA) catheter at the site of occlusion
  - Alteplase (rt-PA):
    - Loading dose: 2-5 mg IA transcatheter delivery
    - Infusion: 1-2 mg/hr by IA transcatheter delivery
- Consult a general surgeon and vascular surgeon early.

→ Serial lactates might not reflect the degree of ischemia; their measurements should be combined with serial abdominal exams.

→ Risk factors for illness include: advanced age, atherosclerosis, atrial fibrillation, congestive heart failure, and hypercoagulability.

→ The gold standard for diagnosis is mesenteric angiography; however, CT angiography is an acceptable initial test.

→ Vasopressors have potential to worsen ischemia and should be used judiciously in patients with persistent hypotension despite adequate volume resuscitation.

→ Treatment varies depending on findings of angiography. Mesenteric arterial embolism and mesenteric arterial thrombosis primarily require surgical management. Mesenteric venous thrombosis and non-occlusive mesenteric ischemia primarily are managed medically.

UPPER GI BLEED
Hemorrhagic/Hypovolemic Shock

Non-variceal UGIB
- Pantoprazole
  - Loading dose: 80 mg IV given over 30 min
  - Infusion: Initiate at 8 mg/hr IV x 72 hrs
- Lansoprazole 60 mg bolus, *THEN* 6 mg/hr x 72 hrs (not available in U.S.)

Massive UGIB with suspected variceal bleed
- Aggressive fluid resuscitation: 0.9% normal saline fluid boluses
- Octreotide
  - Loading dose: 50 mcg (25-100 mcg; usual: 50 mcg) IV
    - Can repeat bolus in first hr if hemorrhage is not controlled.
  - Infusion: 50 mcg/hr (25-50 mcg/hr) IV x 2-5 days
- Somatostatin
  - Loading dose: 250 mcg IV
  - Infusion: 250-500 mcg/hr IV
- *PLUS*
  - Vasopressin
    - Infusion: 0.2-0.4 units/min IV, titrate by doubling dose every 30 min until bleeding stops or MAP >65
    - Max: 0.9 units/min IV
    - Non-surgical candidates (via interventional radiology):
    - Trans-catheter intra-arterial: 0.1-0.5 units/min titrated to effect; taper after 24 hrs
  - Terlipressin *(not available in the U.S.)*
    - Initial dose: 2 mg IV q4 hrs x 48 hrs
    - Maintenance dose: 1 mg IV q4 hrs

Additional therapeutic options and considerations
- Gastric lavage
- Nitroprusside – to counteract excessive HTN, coronary vasospasm, secondary to high-dose vasopressin
  - Infusion: 0.3 mcg/kg/min (usual: 3 mcg/kg/min) IV, titrate 0.5 mcg/kg/min q5 min
    - Max: 10 mcg/kg/min; Onset: 1-2 min; Duration: 1-10 min
    - Avoid using in patients with CrCl <10; doses >3 mcg/kg/min for extended periods of time; can cause thiocyanate toxicity.
- Consider activating massive transfusion protocol (if available) or transfusing 1:1:1 blood products to resuscitate patient in hemorrhagic shock.

→ Consider UGIB if patient's BUN:Cr is >30:1.

→ In cirrhotic patients with UGIB, start antibiotics early (ceftriaxone + ciprofloxacin).

→ A Sengstaken-Blakemore tube can be used for balloon tamponade in the exsanguinating, intubated patient for variceal bleeding when endoscopy is not readily available.

→ Measure lactate levels q2 hrs to evaluate effectiveness of resuscitation.

→ In patients without significant cardiovascular comorbidities or imminent exsanguination, don't transfuse until hemoglobin is less than 7 g/dL to improve outcomes including mortality, especially in patients with suspected variceal bleeding.

ANTICOAGULATION

Class: unfractionated heparin
- **Heparin**
  - Loading dose: 60-80 units/kg IV
    - (max dosing ACS:4,000 units; for PE/VTE max 10,000 units)
  - Maintenance: 12-18 units/kg/hr
  - Monitoring: aPTT target (based on nomogram for underlying diagnosis, but usually 1.5-2.5x control aPTT, can also monitor anti Xa)

Class: low molecular-weight heparin
- **Enoxaparin** (Lovenox)*
  - Loading dose: 1 mg/kg SQ
  - Maintenance: 1 mg/kg SQ q12 hrs *OR* 1.5 mg/kg SQ q24 hrs
  - Monitoring: Anti-Xa levels for patients with renal insufficiency, morbid obesity (>190 kg) or patients who are pregnant
- **Dalteparin** (Fragmin)
  - Dose 200 units/kg SQ q24 hrs *OR* 100 units/kg SQ every 12 hrs
  - Class: glycoprotein IIb/IIIa inhibitor
- **Eptifibatide** (Integrilin)*
  - Loading dose: 180 mcg/kg IV once (max 22.6 kg)
  - Maintenance: 2 mcg/kg/hr (max 15 mg/hr) IV for 18-24 hrs post procedure
  - Note: Reduce dose by 50% in patients with CrCl <50 ml/min.
  - Monitoring: aPTT, ACT
- **Abciximab** (ReoPro)
  - Loading dose: 0.25 mg/kg IV bolus
  - Maintenance: 0.125 mcg/kg/min (max 10 mcg/min) IV for 12 hrs
  - Monitoring: platelets, aPTT, ACT
  - Continue 18-24 hrs in unstable angina.

Class: factor Xa inhibitor
- **Rivaroxaban** (Xarelto)*
  - Loading dose: 15 mg PO bid 3 wks (acute DVT/PE, otherwise none)
  - Dose: 20 mg PO daily
  - Avoid use in patients with CrCl <30 ml/min.
  - Monitoring: none
- **Fondaparinux** (Arixtra)*
  - Dose: <50 kg = 5 mg SQ subcut qday; 50-100 kg= 7.5 mg SQ qday; >100 kg= 10 mg subcut qday
  - Monitoring: Anti-Xa levels (using fondaparinux as calibrator, not commercially available)

- **Apixaban** (not yet approved, but currently under study as VTE treatment)
    - Loading dose: 10 mg PO q12 hrs x 7 days
    - Maintenance dose: 5 mg PO q12 hrs (reduce dosing for elderly, low body weight, renal insufficiency)
    - Avoid in patients with severe renal insufficiency.

Class: Direct Thrombin Inhibitors (DTIs)
- **Bivalirudin** (Angiomax)*
    - **PCI Dosing**
        - Loading dose: 0.75 mg/kg IV once
        - Maintenance: 1.75 mg/kg/hr IV for 4 hrs, **THEN** 0.2 mg/kg/hr IV for up to 20 hrs
        - Monitoring: aPTT, ACT
    - **HIT Dosing**
        - Starting dose: 0.15-0.2 mg/kg/hr
        - Titrate to aPTT 1.5-2.5x control
- **Dabigatran** (Praxada)*
    - Maintenance: 150 mg PO bid
    - Monitoring: none
    - Avoid in patients with severe renal insufficiency (CrCl <30 ml/min).
- **Argatroban**
    - Loading dose: 350 mcg/kg IV bolus
    - Maintenance: 25 mcg/kg/min IV
    - Monitoring: none

Class: Fibrinolytics
- **Alteplase (rt-PA)**
    - **PE:** 10 mg IV bolus, **THEN** 90 mg IV infusion over 2 hrs
    - **STEMI:** 15 mg IV bolus, **THEN** 0.75 mg/kg over 30 min, **THEN** 0.5 mg/kg over 60 min (max 100 mg)
    - **CVA:** total dose 0.9 mg/kg; load 10% of total dose over 1 min, **THEN** give remaining 90% IV over 60 mins
        - Monitoring: neurologic and BP checks

*Indicates renal dosing is required if creatinine clearance is impaired.

Pearls
→ Avoid argatroban, rivaroxaban, apixaban, and dabigatran in patients with hepatic impairment.
→ Consider synthetic Factor Xa inhibitor or DTIs in patients with a history of heparin-induced thrombocytopenia (HIT).
→ Clinical coagulation measures can be altered by non-monitored anticoagulants (rivaroxaban, apixaban, dabigatran), but do not accurately reflect effect.
→ No consensus exists on alteplase use in cardiac arrest with suspected PE.
→ Refer to individual chapters for contraindications to fibrinolytic therapy.

ANTICOAGULATION REVERSAL

- **Warfarin (Coumadin)** – Inhibits vitamin K-dependent clotting factors (II, VII, IX, X).
    - *See Table 3 for current ACCP guideline-based recommendations.*
    - Vitamin K_1 (phytonadione)
        - PO dose: 1-5 mg
            - Onset: 6-10 hrs; Peak effect: 24-48 hrs
        - IV dose: 5-10 mg, slow infusion of diluted solution ($\geq$50 mL) over at least 20 min
            - Onset: 1-2 hrs; Peak effect: 12-14 hrs
            - Risk of anaphylaxis ~3:10,000 doses
    - Fresh frozen plasma (FFP)
        - Dose: 10-30 mL/kg or 2-4 units IV, repeat as needed
        - Onset: 2-6 hrs
            - Max INR reduction to 1.4
    - Prothrombin complex concentrate (PCC)
        - Faster infusion than FFP; low volume makes PCC useful in patients where volume status is a concern (e.g., CHF).
        - Risk of heparin-induced thrombocytopenia (HIT) as some products contain heparin.
        - 3-Factor (Bebulin VH, Profilnine SD) non-activated PCC (factors II, IX, X; factor VII low-negligible content)
            - Dose: 25-50 IU/kg slow IV; max rate: 2 mL/min (Bebulin VH), 10 mL/min (Profilnine SD)
                - INR based dosing: INR <5: 30 IU/kg, INR>5: 50 IU/kg
                - Repeat for INR >1.2
            - Onset: <30 min
            - Bebulin VH contains heparin and natural rubber/latex. Profilnine SD does not contain heparin.
            - If using 3-factor PCCs, give 1-2 units of FFP for factor VII replacement.
        - 4-Factor (Kcentra, US; non-activated PCC (Factors II, VII, IX, and X)
            - INR based dosing: INR 2 to <4: 25 units/kg (max 2500 units); INR 4-6: 35 units/kg (max 3500 units); INR >6: 50 units/kg (max 5000 units)
            - Contains heparin.
            - Administer with vitamin K concurrently.
- **Aspirin/clopidogrel (Plavix)/prasugrel (Effient)** – prevent platelet aggregation (ASA inhibits thromboxane A2 formation); clopidogrel/prasugrel block ADP platelet receptor; ticagrelor (Brillinta) P2Y12 allosteric antagonists
    - Platelet transfusion (unproven, but generally accepted reversal)
        - Dose: 1 apheresed unit or 5-10 "packs" of random donor platelets, repeat as needed
            - 6-pack of platelets is about 1 apheresed unit (single donor)

- **Unfractionated heparin** – potentiates antithrombin III, prevents fibrinogen conversion to fibrin
  - Protamine sulfate
    - Dose: 1 mg slow IV per 100 units of heparin used in last 2-3 hrs; max dose: 50 mg
      - Lower dose if time elapsed since heparin infused:
        - If 30-60 min elapsed: 0.5-0.75 mg per 100 units of heparin
        - If >2 hrs elapsed: 0.25-0.375 mg per 100 units of heparin
    - Max infusion rate: 50 mg/10 min; can cause histamine release/anaphylactoid reaction.
- **Low molecular-weight heparins** (LMWH) (e.g., enoxaparin [Lovenox], dalteparin [Fragmin]); inhibit factor Xa and factor IIa (thrombin)
  - Protamine sulfate
    - Partial reversal only: anti-Xa activity is not completely neutralized.
    - Initial dose: 1 mg slow IV per 1 mg of enoxaparin, **OR** each 100 anti-Xa units of dalteparin; if LMWH given within the past 8 hrs; max dose 50 mg
    - Repeat dose if bleeding continues or aPTT remains prolonged 2-4 hrs after first dose.
      - Give 0.5 mg slow IV per 1 mg of enoxaparin, or each 100 anti-Xa units of dalteparin.
    - Max infusion rate: 50 mg/10 min; can cause histamine release/anaphylactoid reaction.
- **Dabigatran (Pradaxa)** – direct thrombin inhibitor
  - No specific antidote. No reliable lab values to trend. aPTT possibly for qualitative assessment, but curvilinear relationship limits interpretation. TT increases linearly, but strength of correlation reduced at higher concentrations.
  - Protamine and vitamin K1 are NOT expected to be useful.
  - *Consider:* **hemodialysis/CVVHD**, FFP, rFVIIa, PCC, charcoal if ≤2 hrs after ingestion.
  - Note: Dialysis will remove approximately 60% of active dabigatran.
- **Rivaroxaban (Xarelto), Apixaban (Eliquis)** – direct factor Xa inhibitors
  - No specific antidote. PT increases linearly, but is not sensitive at near normal PT values. aPTT should NOT be used be used to assess coagulability.
  - Consider: FFP; PCC 25 units/kg IBW IV over 10 min, may repeat x1 (rivaroxaban); charcoal for last rivaroxaban dose <2 hr or last apixaban dose <6 hours.
  - Rivaroxaban and apixaban are NOT dialyzable.
- **Thrombolytics** (e.g., rt-PA [alteplase], streptokinase): activates plasmin to lyse clots
  - Cryoprecipitate: 10 units IV
  - Aminocaproic acid: 4-5 g IV in 250 mL over 60 min, **THEN** 1 g/hr until hemostasis
    - Reserve for life-threatening bleed; contraindicated in DIC; max 30 g/day.
  - *Consider:* FFP (2-4 units), platelets (5-10 random donor)

- **Glycoprotein IIb-IIIa inhibitors** – inhibits platelet aggregation
    - Abciximab (ReoPro), eptifibatide (Integrillin), tirofiban (AggraStat)
        - Abciximab half life ~12 hours; others are ~4 hours
        - Reversal with non-affected platelets
            - 1 unit aphereseed or 5-10 packs of donor platelets as needed

Table 3: Coumadin Reversal Recommendations		
INR	Bleeding	Action
4.5 – 10	Without bleeding	No vitamin K
>10	Without bleeding	PO Vitamin K
Any	Major bleeding	IV 4-Factor PCC, rather than FFP PLUS Vitamin K 5-10 mg IV

Adapted from the 9th ACCP guidelines for anticoagulation/warfarin (Vitamin K antagonists) reversal.

PEARLS

→ Obtain type and screen early; type and crossmatch if use of blood products is anticipated.
→ Infuse vitamin K slowly and watch for anaphylaxis.
→ Protamine should be administered no faster than 50 mg/10 min to avoid hypotension and cardiovascular collapse; excess dose may result in anticoagulation.
→ During massive transfusions, remember to replace clotting factors, platelets, and calcium (pRBCs:FFP:platelets is 1:1:1).
→ Consider 4-factor PCC for patients with massive bleeding who are taking an oral anticoagulant.

COAGULOPATHY REVERSAL

- **Hemophilia A** (↓ Factor VIII); Lab Findings:↑ aPTT
  - *Recombinant factor VIII*
    - Est. dose of Factor VIII (IU) = Weight (kg) x (Desired % increase) x 0.5
      - In an emergency, assume level of Factor VIII is zero.
      - Initial dose of 50 IU/kg IV provides 100% replacement.
    - Half-life: 8-12 hours
    - Severe bleeding (ICH, trauma, major surgery):
      - 50 IU/kg IV loading dose (100%), ***THEN*** keep at least 50% replacement with subsequent dosing (25-50 IU/kg) IV q6-12 hrs.
      - May consider continuous infusion of 2-4 IU/kg/hr to maintain levels obtained after initial bolus.
    - Moderate bleeding: (e.g., bleeding that requires blood transfusion, but does not result in hemodynamic instability):
      - May need only 1-2 doses of 25-50 IU/kg IV q 8-12 hrs.
    - Mild bleeding
      - 15-20 IU/kg IV; may consider supplement with tranexamic acid (TXA) ***OR*** aminocaproic acid (especially for mucocutaneous bleeding) ***OR*** DDAVP alone (see below).
  - *Additional therapeutic options and considerations*
    - Recombinant Factor VII (Novo Seven): 90-120 mcg/kg q2 hrs IV until hemostatic
    - Cryoprecipitate: 1 unit/10kg IV
    - Fresh frozen plasma (FFP): 15-20 mL/kg IV
    - Tranexamic acid: 25-50 mg/kg/day; max 4 g; divided into 3-4 PO or IV doses
    - Aminocaproic acid: 50-100 mg/kg PO/IV (max 5 g) over 30-60 min; ***THEN*** 1-4 g q 4-8 hours (max 30 g/day)
    - Desmopressin (DDAVP): 0.3 mcg/kg in 50 mL NS IV over 20 min (may also be given IM or intranasal (high-concentration nasal spray)
    - PCC: not routinely recommended given expense, unpredictable action, short half-life and thrombotic risks.
- **Hemophilia B** (↓ Factor IX); Lab findings: ↑ aPTT
  - *Recombinant factor IX*
    - Initial dose: 100 IU/kg IV corresponds to 100% replacement
      - Half-life: 16-17 hrs
  - *Additional options similar to those for hemophilia A, except:*
    - DDAVP is **not** recommended because of the risk of inducing thrombocytopenia.
    - If using TXA or aminocaproic acid, use purified Factor IX to avoid thrombotic risks.

- **VonWillebrand Disease:** ↑ aPTT, ↑ bleeding time; platelets may be decreased or normal (although impaired in functioning).
  - *Type 1 or 2:*
    - DDAVP: 0.3 mcg/kg in 50 mL NS IV over 20 min
    - Highly purified VWF concentrate (HPVWF, brands: Humate-P or Wilate)
      - Humate-P: loading dose of 60-80 units/kg IV, ***THEN*** 40-60 units IV q8-12 hrs x 3 days
      - Wilate: loading dose of 40-60 units/kg IV, ***THEN*** 20-40 units IV q12-24 hrs x 5-7 days
      - *Consider if DDAVP is ineffective.*
    - *Type 2b:* Cannot be treated with DDAVP as it may worsen symptoms, unless patient is known to have tolerated it or undergoes trial infusion first.
  - *Type 3:* HPVWF, Factor VIII, cryoprecipitate
    - Cannot be treated with DDAVP as this type is not likely to respond.
  - Additional treatment for severe bleeding: Recombinant factor VIII, cryoprecipitate
- **Disseminated intravascular coagulation (DIC):** ↓ fibrinogen/platelets, ↑ d-dimer/PT/aPTT
  - Underlying cause (sepsis, trauma, obstetrical emergencies) **MUST** be treated.
  - Use FFP, platelet transfusion, cryoprecipitate, vitamin K as temporizing measures for patients who are bleeding or at high risk for bleeding.
    - Goal: Platelets >50 k, fibrinogen >150 mg/dL
  - Paradoxical concurrent hypercoaguability (e.g., VTE); consider low-dose heparin infusion (300-500 units/hr) without bolus.
    - There is only Grade C/Level IV evidence for this, and regimens vary.
- **Thrombotic thrombocytopenic purpura/ (TTP):** ↓ platelets, anemia, normal PT/ aPTT, + schistocytes on peripheral blood smear
  - Spectrum of hemolytic uremic syndrome (HUS)
  - Treat with therapeutic plasma exchange.
    - ***PLUS*** methylprednisolone (125 mg IV bid) ***OR*** prednisone (1 mg/kg QD)
    - While plasma exchange is recommended, plasma infusion can also be used emergently.
  - Goal platelets >10,000
- **Idiopathic thrombocytopenic purpura (ITP):** ↓ platelets, ↑ bleeding time
  - ***NB:*** guidelines vary when treating children
  - Platelet transfusion for <30k or severe bleeding
  - Initial treatment: Prednisone (1 mg/kg/day PO) or high-dose dexamethasone (40 mg/day PO or IV)
  - Resistant or severe disease:
    - Methylprednisolone (30 mg/kg IV x 3 days; then tapered)
    - IVIG (1 g/kg/day x 1-2 days)

- If patient is Rh (+), anti-D antibody (Rhophylac, Win Rho; 50 mcg/kg IV over 3-5 min).
  - "Black box" warning exists for severe hemolysis with anti-D administration; therefore, avoid its use in patients with bleeding or evidence of autoimmune hemolysis.
  - Consider reduced dose (25-40 mcg/kg) if Hgb <10 g/dL; use alternative if Hgb<8 g/dL.
- Many patients ultimately require therapeutic splenectomy.
- **Liver disease:** Platelets ↓, PT, aPTT ↔/↑
  - With chronic liver disease, no need to treat prolonged coagulation times in the absence of bleeding.
  - For active bleeding PRBC (>7 g/dL): FFP (10-20 ml/kg), platelets (1 unit increases PLT ~5k-8k; goal >50 k), vitamin K (5 mg PO or 5-10 mg IV over 1 hour)
    - PO Vitamin K preferred given risk for anaphylaxis with IV preparation
  - Temporizing measure in liver failure
- **Renal disease:** Platelets ↔/↑, bleeding time ↑
  - DDAVP: 0.3 mcg/kg IV infused over 10 min
  - Dialysis
- **Heparin-induced thrombocytopenia (HIT):** ↓ Platelets
  - Type I (most common, no clinical significance) or Type II (immune-mediated thrombosis)
  - Risks: Long duration of therapy, UFH, surgical patients, females
  - Use the "4T" clinical pretest score to determine further testing.
    - ELISA test is first line; functional assay is second line; SRA is the gold standard for confirmation.
  - Treat by IMMEDIATELY stopping all forms of heparin.
    - Start non-heparin anticoagulant (e.g., Argatroban)
  - Patients with documented HIT with thrombosis need long-term anticoagulation.
- **Thrombocytopenia** (other causes)
  - Alcoholism, medication-induced (antibiotics, antiepileptics, chemotherapy, etc.), splenic sequestration, SLE, HIV, HELLP (hemolysis, elevated liver enzymes, low platelets [seen in pregnancy]), malignancy, leukemia, lymphoma
  - Platelets are rarely needed unless <10,000 or in the setting of trauma/bleeding.

PEARLS

→ Obtain type and screen early; type and cross-match if use of blood products is anticipated.
→ If patient is transplant/BMT candidate, have blood products leuko-reduced, CMV safe and irradiated.
→ In DIC, treating the underlying cause has priority over correcting lab values.
→ Consider patient's coagulation status before performing invasive procedures.

TUMOR LYSIS SYNDROME

Treatment

- Laboratory monitoring (BMP, mag, phos, LDH, uric acid) q6 hours
- Fluid resuscitation
  - Loading: 0.9% NaCl (normal saline) or other isotonic IV fluid bolus x1-2 L
  - Maintenance infusion: 200-250 mL/hour
  - Goal urine output: 2 mL/kg/hr
- Hyperuricemia
  - Allopurinol:
    - Will only decrease production of uric acid, but not clear hyperuricemia so should be used only as prophylaxis.
    - Dosing
      - Up to 800 mg PO divided bid to qid with food and plenty fluids.
        - ◆ Adjust for renal insufficiency.
        - ◆ Doses greater than 300 mg should be divided.
  - Rasburicase:
    - Dosing
      - High risk or uric acid >7.5 mg/dL: 0.2 mg/kg IV daily
      - Intermediate risk with uric acid <7.5 mg/dL: 0.15 mg/kg IV daily
      - Low risk with uric acid <7.5 mg/dL: 0.1 mg/kg IV daily
      - Limited data: Single dose 3 mg or 6 mg effective at rapidly lowering uric acid
    - Contraindicated in patients with G6PD deficiency, pregnant, or lactating women.
    - Duration of therapy 1-7 days (average: 2 days)
- Hyperkalemia
  - Calcium gluconate (10%): 3 amps (30 ml) IV at 1.5 mL/min (peripheral IV) *OR* calcium chloride (10%) IV 1 amp (10 ml) (central line)
  - Regular insulin 10 units IV concurrent with 1-2 amps 50% dextrose (D50)
  - Temporize with high dose nebulized albuterol 10-20 mg
- Phosphate binders
  - Aluminum hydroxide 50-100 mg/kg/day PO divided q6 hrs x 1-2 days

Additional therapeutic options and considerations

- Foley catheter for urine output monitoring
- Hemodialysis in patients with poor urine output, worsening renal function, or refractory hyperkalemia
- Urinary alkalinization is controversial and should not be routinely performed. It may increase calcium-phosphate crystal formation; it may be beneficial with very high uric acid levels and normal phosphate.
  - Sodium bicarbonate (8.4%): 1-2 amp bolus *OR* add 1-3 amps to D_5W infusion
  - Goal urine pH 6.5-7.5

Pearls

→ Consider febuxostat, a novel xanthine oxidase inhibitor, if allopurinol contraindicated.

→ Consider tumor lysis syndrome in cancer patients with ECG changes, renal failure, or mental status changes, especially in setting of recent chemotherapy.

→ Due to effectiveness of rasburicase and high phosphate within malignant cells, calcium-phosphate crystallization is becoming leading cause of renal failure.

→ Extent of mortality directly related to degree of renal involvement.

ANAPHYLAXIS

Treatment

- Epinephrine: (1:1000) 0.01 mg/kg IM (usual adult dose is 0.2-0.5 mg)
    - May be repeated q5-10 min
    - Epipen/Twinject: 0.3 mg IM/SQ injection
- Epinephrine: 0.1 mg (1:10,000) IV given over 5 min
- Fluid resuscitation: start with 1-2 liters of 0.9% normal saline IV (bolus); may need several liters.
- If patient is persistently hypotensive (MAP <65)
    - Epinephrine
        - Infusion: 1-2 mcg/min IV, titrate by 1 mcg/min q10 min
        - Max: none (suggested max 0.5 mcg/kg/min); Onset: 1-2 min
    - There is no clear superiority of other pressors in refractory anaphylaxis alone or when added to epinephrine; however, vasopressin, 0.01-0.04 units/min, has been reported effective in several cases.
- Adjunctive treatment
    - Antihistamines
        - H1 antagonist:
            - Diphenhydramine: 50 mg IV q6 hrs x 48-72 hrs
        - H2 antagonist:
            - Famotidine: 20 mg IV bid x 48-72 hrs
            - Ranitidine: 50 mg IV q6 hrs x 48-72 hrs
            - Cimetidine: 300 mg IV q6 hrs x 48-72 hrs
    - Corticosteroids
        - Methylprednisolone: 60-125 mg IV q6-q24 hrs
        - Hydrocortisone: 5 mg/kg IV q4-6 hrs (250-500 mg)

Additional therapeutic options and considerations

- Albuterol: 2.5 mg INH q20 min PRN bronchospasm

PEARLS

→ Prompt administration of epinephrine is the only intervention proven to improve mortality in patients with anaphylactic shock.

→ IM injection of epinephrine provides superior absorption profiles compared with subcutaneous injection; the preferred site of injection is the lateral thigh.

→ If epinephrine drip is not immediately available, add 1 mL of 1:1000 **OR** 10 mL of 1:10,000 epinephrine to a 1L bag of NS to make a 1 mcg/mL solution. Start at 1 mL/ min =1 mcg/min and titrate.

→ Clinical course can be biphasic, with a second reaction occurring up to 72 hrs later, despite no further exposures to the trigger.

- In pregnant patients with anaphylaxis, treat with the same interventions. In addition, administer 100% O2, place in left lateral decubitus, maintain SBP >90, and monitor the fetus.
- There is growing evidence in the literature suggesting earlier consideration of using methylene blue for refractory anaphylactic shock, but it has yet to be added to the *World Allergy Organization Anaphylaxis Guidelines*.

ECLAMPSIA

New-onset HTN[1]	Proteinuria[2]	AKI3, pulmonary edema, RUQ pain, cerebral or visual Δs	↑↑↑LFTs or low platelets[4]	Hemolysis[5]	Seizure
Pre-eclampsia					
		Severe pre-eclampsia[5]			
				HELLP syndrome	
		Eclampsia			

Shaded areas are features that may be present in each syndrome, but are not required for the diagnosis.

1. New-onset hypertension in a woman ≥20 weeks pregnant is defined
   Pre-eclampsia:
   SBP >160 or DBP >110 on a single measure, or
   SBP >140 or DBP >90 on two measures, 4 hrs apart
   Severe pre-eclampsia:
   SBP >160 or DBP >110 on two measures, 4 hrs apart
2. Urine dip 1+, ≥300 mg/24 hour urine, or protein/creatinine ratio ≥0.3
3. Cr ≥1.1 mg/dL or an unexplained doubling of baseline creatinine
4. Liver function tests at ≥2x upper limit normal, or platelet count <100,000 microliter
5. Seizure + pre-eclampsia with any, some, or none of the above features

Treatment

- **Seizure prevention and treatment**
  - Magnesium sulfate
    - Loading dose: 4-6 gm IV over 15-20 min
    - Infusion: 2 gm/hr; Duration: 24 hours after last seizure
      - May re-bolus with 2 gm if seizure recurs
    - Max: 40 gm/24 hrs
- **Blood pressure management**
  - Goal: SBP <160 mmHg **AND** DBP <105 mmHg
  - Hydralazine
    - Initial dosing: 5-10 mg IV q15-20 min to goal
    - Max: 40 mg/dose; Onset: 5-20 min; Duration: 1-4 hrs
  - Labetalol
    - Loading dose: 20 mg IV, double dose at 10-min intervals to max of 80 mg
    - Infusion: 2-8 mg/min, titrate by 0.5 mg/min q10 min
    - Max: 8 mg/min; Onset: 2-5 min; Duration 2-4 hrs
      - *Note: Consider alternative agents if blood pressure is refractory to high doses of labetalol.*

- Nicardipine
    - Infusion: 5 mg/hr IV, increase by 2.5 mg/hr q5-15 min
    - Max: 15 mg/hr; Onset: 1-2 min; Duration: 40 min
- **Delivery**
    - Patients with severe pre-eclampsia and eclampsia should be medically stabilized, then delivered in a timely fashion.
    - Method is dependent on maternal factors and should be done in a tertiary center.

PEARLS

→ Always consider eclampsia in a seizing woman of child-bearing age.

→ Eclamptic seizures occur in the antepartum (50%), intrapartum (25%), and postpartum periods (25%).

→ Earliest sign of magnesium toxicity is depressed reflexes, followed by respiratory depression.

→ Treat severe magnesium toxicity with IV calcium.

→ The FDA considers magnesium sulfate Pregnancy Category D because IV infusions longer than 5-7 days in duration may result in fetal osteopenia and bone growth abnormalities.

→ The diagnostic criteria for pre-eclampsia, severe pre-eclampsia, and eclampsia have changed.

PULMONARY HYPERTENSION (PH)
Obstructive, Cardiogenic Shock

Definition: PA mean pressure >25 mmHg at rest, measured by right heart catheterization; acute decompensated RV failure with increased PA pressure.

Treatment
Precipitating factors
- Empiric treatment for bacteremia is warranted in these patients who often have chronic indwelling intravenous catheters.
- Perform cardioversion in patients with tachyarrhythmias; if this is not possible, rate control with digoxin or amiodarone (avoid beta blockers or verapamil).
- Bradycardias may require temporary pacing.

Hypoxemia
- Avoid hypoxemia and hypercarbia, as they are both vasoconstrictors.
- Liberal oxygen administration
  - Goal SpO_2 >90-92%
- If mechanical ventilation is absolutely necessary, employ the lowest plateau pressures through low tidal volume and low PEEP.
  - Avoid permissive hypercapnia.
- Aggressively manage bronchospasm and agitation.

Hypotension
- Rapid assessment of volume status with CVP, PA catheter, or echocardiography
  - If CVP <5 mmHg, cautious volume challenges of crystalloid with a goal of 10 to 12 mmHg; if no response, consider early vasopressor therapy.
  - Alternately, a 250 mL NS or plasmalyte fluid challenge may be given; if no response, consider early vasopressor therapy.
  - Norepinephrine
    - Infusion: 0.05 mcg/kg/min IV, titrate by 0.02 mcg/kg/min q 5 min
    - Dose range: 0.05-0.5 mcg/kg/min; Onset: 1-2 min; Duration: 1-2 min
    - No true max, but consider using additional agents if patient is unresponsive to higher doses.

Pulmonary vasodilators
- Inhaled agents:
  - Nitric oxide inhaled (INO): start at 20 ppm, increase to max of 40 ppm
    - Before starting, obtain ABG and methemoglobin level (q6 hrs).
    - Rebound PH can occur with brief interruptions.
  - Epoprostenol inhaled (Flolan): 5000 to 20000 ng/mL as a continuous nebulization
    - Causes systemic effects, unlike INO.
- If not hypotensive, intravenous epoprostenol or oral sildenafil
  - Epoprostenol (Flolan/Veletri) infusion: 1-2 ng/kg/min IV, titrate by 1-2 ng/kg/min q15-30 min until dose-limiting effects are elicited or no further improvement.
    - Dose-limiting effects include: hypotension, headache, flushing, jaw pain, nausea/vomiting, abdominal pain, diarrhea, myalgias, and arthralgias.

Inotropic support
- Add an inotrope in normotensive patients with persistently elevated serum lactate level, SvO_2 <65% or $ScvO_2$ <70% despite previous treatments.
  - Dobutamine
    - Infusion: 2.5 mcg/kg/min IV, titrate by 2.5 mcg/kg/min q 10 min
    - Max: 20 mcg/kg/min; Onset: 1-10 min; Duration: 10 min
  - Milrinone
    - Loading dose: 50 mcg/kg IV over 10 min
    - Infusion: 0.375 mcg/kg/min IV, titrate by 0.005 mcg/kg/min q 5-10 min
    - Max: 0.75 mcg/kg/min; Onset: 5-15 min; Duration: 3-5 hrs
    - *Note: Milrinone's duration of action is prolonged in patients with renal insufficiency.*

Mechanical circulatory support
- For refractory shock, consider RV assist devices/VA ECMO/pumpless lung assist devices, pulmonary thromboendarterectomy, atrial septostomy, or lung transplantation/heart-lung transplantation.

After stabilization
- Diuresis
  - Loop diuretic (e.g., furosemide) by IV bolus or continuous infusion (the latter is associated with constant diuresis and decreased ototoxicity)
    - Intermittent bolus dose: 20-80 mg IV bolus
    - Loading dose: 20-40 mg IV over 1-2 min
    - Infusion: 5 mg/hr, titrate by 5-20 mg/hr to a max of 160 mg/hr
  - If loop diuretic is insufficient, add a thiazide diuretic (e.g., chlorothiazide IV or PO, or metolazone PO).
  - If no hyperkalemia, spironolactone can be added.
- Consider CVVHD if patient fails medical management.
- Transition to chronic pulmonary vasodilator when possible.

PEARLS

→ **Do not turn off or remove the pump** in those patients receiving continuous medications with a very short half-life (epoprostenol IV, treprostinil SQ/IV). Acute discontinuation can result in life-threatening rebound pulmonary hypertension.

→ Vasodilator therapy is not without risks; it can cause systemic hypotension or worsen PH. If the pulmonary artery diameter is fixed, it will just cause decreased right heart pressures without affecting pulmonary vasculature.

→ Right ventricular failure is a hallmark finding with decompensated PH.

→ Patients with Group I pulmonary arterial hypertension (PAH) are most likely on chronic warfarin with goal INR 1.5-2.5.

PULMONARY EMBOLISM (PE)

Anticoagulation
- Unfractionated heparin (UFH)
    - Initial bolus: 80 units/kg IV
    - Infusion: 18 units/kg/hr IV; titrate q6 hrs to goal aPTT (1.5-2.5x control)
- Low molecular-weight heparin (LMWH)
    - Enoxaparin: 1 mg/kg subcutaneously q12 hours (if CrCl ≥30 ml/min)
- Fondaparinux
    - Administer subcutaneously; discontinue if platelet count <100K.
    - Dose: <50 kg: 5 mg, 50-100 kg: 7.5 mg, >100 kg: 10 mg
- Warfarin PO: titrate to INR 2-3; begin after UFH or LMWH initiated then overlap for at least 5 days and until INR ≥2 for at least 24 hrs.
- New oral anticoagulants
    - Rivaroxaban 15 mg PO twice daily for 21 days followed by 20 mg PO once daily
        - Factor Xa inhibitor; avoid if CrCl <30 ml/min
        - No specific antidote/reversal agent available.

Massive PE (Defined as PE with SBP <90 for >15 min)
- Fibrinolytics
    - Alteplase *(fibrinolytic of choice in the U.S.)*
        - Initial dose: 10 mg IV bolus
        - Infusion: 90 mg IV over 2 hrs
    - Streptokinase *(most widely available option outside of the U.S.)*
        - Initial dose: 250,000 units IV over 30 min
        - Infusion: 100,000 units/hr IV for 12-24 hrs
    - Tenecteplase *(non-labeled use)*
        - Dose: <60 kg: 30 mg; 60-69 kg: 35 mg; 70-79 kg: 40 mg; 80-89 kg: 45 mg; >90 kg: 50 mg; given IV bolus over 5-10 seconds
    - See Table 4 for contraindications.

Submassive PE
- Consider fibrinolytic therapy in submassive PE if:
    - Intermittent hypotension
    - Respiratory failure
    - Moderate/severe right ventricular strain
        - RV hypokinesis or dilation, estimated RVSP >40 mmHg, McConnell's sign
    - Elevated biomarkers (i.e., BNP, pro-BNP, troponin)
    - See Table 4 for contraindications.
- MOPETT study: "safe dose" alteplase (plus UFH **OR** LMWH) improved PAPs at 28 days with no difference in mortality or bleeding
    - If ≥50 kg, give 50 mg (10 mg bolus over 10 min; remaining 40 mg over 2 hrs)
    - If <50 kg, give 0.5 mg/kg (10 mg bolus over 10 min; remaining dose over 2 hrs)
- PEITHO study: tenecteplase (full dose) plus UFH improved primary outcome (composite of mortality or hemodynamic collapse at 7 days) with 8% major bleeding

- A recent study showed that "safe dose" alteplase (see above) plus oral rivaroxaban in 98 patients with moderate (n=84) and severe (n=14) PE improved PA pressures at 28 days. UFH and rivaroxaban regimens were modified.

Blood pressure management: target MAP >70

- Fluid resuscitation: 0.9% NaCl (normal saline): 250-500 mL IV bolus *(see Pearls Section)*
- Vasopressors
  - Norepinephrine
    - Infusion: 0.05 mcg/kg/min IV, titrate by 0.02 mcg/kg/min q5 min
    - Dose range: 0.05-0.5 mcg/kg/min; Onset: 1-2 min; Duration: 1-2 min
    - No true max, but consider using additional agents if patient is unresponsive to higher doses.
  - Inotropes
    - Dobutamine may be used in combination with a vasopressor to augment cardiac contractility; may cause hypotension when used alone.
      - Infusion: 2.5 mcg/kg/min IV, titrate by 2.5 mcg/kg/min q10 min
      - Max: 20 mcg/kg/min; Onset: 1-2 min; Duration: 10 min

Table 4: Contraindications to Fibrinolytics in PE
Absolute contraindications
• History of intracranial hemorrhage • Active bleeding (menstruation is NOT a contraindication)
Relative contraindications
• Known intracranial neoplasm, AVM, or aneurysm • Significant head trauma within the past 15 days • Intracranial or intra-spinal surgery within the past 3 months • Cerebrovascular accident within the past 2 months • Recent surgery or organ biopsy • Recent trauma (within the past 15 days) • Venipuncture at a non-compressible site • Uncontrolled hypertension (SBP >180 mmHg, DBP >110 mmHg) • Recent GI or internal bleeding (within past 10 days) • Known bleeding diathesis • Significant hepatic or renal impairment • Pregnancy

Refer to American College of Chest Physician Guidelines for comprehensive list of contraindications (http://www.chestnet.org/Guidelines-and-Resources/Guidelines-and-Consensus-Statements/Antithrombotic-Guidelines-9th-Ed).

PEARLS

→ Avoid aggressive fluid administration, which can lead to RV over-distension and worsen RV failure.

→ Catheter-based intervention or embolectomy may be considered for systemic fibrinolytic failure, or when contraindication to systemic fibrinolysis exists.

→ Therapeutic aPTT ranges differ among institutions; consult local protocols.
→ Monitor anti-Xa levels with LMWH use in: obese, low body weight, elderly and renal-insufficient patients.
→ In the U.S., pausing the heparin infusion is recommended during fibrinolytic infusion.
→ Consider fibrinolytics in cardiac arrest due to suspected PE (but not for undifferentiated arrest).

STATUS ASTHMATICUS

Treatment

- Oxygen therapy: goal SpO_2 >90%, >95% for patients who are pregnant or with significant heart disease.
- Inhaled β_2 agonists:
  - Albuterol (first line):
    - Continuous nebulization: 10-15 mg/hr INH
    - Intermittent:
      - Nebulized solution: 2.5-5 mg INH q20 min x 3 doses, **THEN** 2.5-10 mg q1-4 hrs PRN
      - MDI + spacer: 4-8 puffs INH q20 min (up to 4 hrs), **THEN** q1-4 hrs PRN
- Inhaled anticholinergics:
  - Ipratropium bromide:
    - Nebulized solution: 0.5 mg INH q20 min x 3 doses, **THEN** PRN wheezing
    - MDI: 8 puffs INH q20 min PRN up to 3 hrs
- Glucocorticoids:
  - Methylprednisolone: 1 mg/kg IV/PO x 1 (Max: 80 mg)
  - Prednisone/prednisolone: 1 mg/kg PO x 1 (Max: 80 mg)
  - Anti-inflammatory onset in 4-6 hrs; IV and PO efficacy are the same.
- IV fluid resuscitation with crystalloid solution

Additional therapeutic options and considerations

- Improve ventilation, reduce work of breathing.
  - Bronchodilation
    - Magnesium: 2 g IV over 20 min (if after 1 hour of conventional therapy fails)
      - Use with caution in patients with renal insufficiency; side effect of muscle weakness, respiratory depression, hypotension.
    - Nonselective β-agonists: Consider one if patient is in extremis or if initial inhaled β agonists fail. Do NOT use both concurrently.
      - Terbutaline: 0.25 mg SQ, may repeat q20 min x 3 doses, max 0.75 mg in 1-hr period.
      - Epinephrine: 0.3-0.5 mg [of a 1:100 (1 mg/ml) concentration] SQ, q20 min (up to 3 doses)
        - Side effects include myocardial irritability, dysrhythmias, and nervousness.

- - - ◆ Use caution if patient is >40 or has coronary artery disease, but there is no absolute contraindication.
  - ▪ Theophylline: *No longer recommended due to no additional bronchodilation above that provided by β-agonists without increased adverse side effects.*
    - • Loading dose no longer indicated
    - • Initial dose: 0.4 mg/kg/hr (max 900 mg/24 hr)
    - • Adjust maintenance dose:
      - ◆ 0.2 mg/kg/hr if patient has liver disease, cor pulmonale, or cardiac decompensation
      - ◆ 0.3 mg/kg/hr if patient is >60 years old (max 400 mg/24 hr)
      - ◆ 0.7 mg/kg/hr in smokers
    - • Determine presence of major drug interactions requiring preemptive dose adjustment. Use IBW to calculate dose. Therapeutic range: 10-15 mcg/mL.
    - • Obtain baseline level if patient is on long-term administration and after initiating IV.
    - • Contraindicated with corn/corn product allergy.
- • Improve oxygenation
  - – Heliox: decreases airway resistance by increasing laminar flow; more helpful in peds. Consider using in conjunction with albuterol nebs in severe cases.
    - ▪ Dose: 70:30 helium:oxygen, but can use 60-80% helium
- • Intubation/induction
  - – Ketamine: dissociative, bronchodilation, anxiolysis, min respiratory depression
    - ▪ Induction dose: 1-2 mg/kg IV bolus
    - ▪ Continuous infusion: Initiate at 0.5 mg/kg/hr IV
    - ▪ Side effects include: laryngospasm, emergence reactions, hypertension, myoclonus, hypersalivation
    - ▪ For hypersalivation, consider the following:
      - • Glycopyrrolate: 0.1 mg IV q2-3 min PRN, *OR*
      - • Atropine: 0.4-0.6 mg IV/IM/SQ q4-6 hrs PRN
- **• In refractory cases, consider inhalational anesthetics or ECMO under expert consultation.**

PEARLS

→ Mechanical ventilation should be a last resort, as it places patients at very high risk of pneumothorax, pneumomediastinum, worsening bronchospasm, and hypotension.
→ High dose β-agonists administration can cause lactic acidosis.
→ Watch for autopeep/breathstacking if patient on a ventilator.
→ Treat pregnant women aggressively, as respiratory acidosis is harmful to fetus.
→ Look for occult infection (i.e., sinus infection) as trigger in compliant patients.
→ Monitor serum potassium in patients requiring continuous albuterol nebulizer treatments.

SEPTIC SHOCK

Distributive Shock

- **Volume resuscitation**
  - Initial crystalloid infusion (preferentially LR or chloride-restrictive solution)
    - Minimum 30 mL/kg initial bolus **OR** 500 mL boluses with frequent monitoring of perfusion indices
    - Goal-directed resuscitation in first 6 hrs: MAP >65, urine output >0.5 mL/kg/hr, ScvO$_2$ >70% **OR** mixed SvO$_2$ >65%, and rapid lactate normalization
  - **Consider** addition of albumin (5%): boluses of 250-500 mL.
  - Look for signs of volume responsiveness with dynamic (pulse pressure variation, stroke volume variation), static measurements (arterial pressure, heart rate), IVC collapsibility, or passive leg raise test.
- **Vasopressors: Goal MAP >65**
  - *First-line pressors*
    - Norepinephrine *(first choice)*
      - Infusion: 0.05 mcg/kg/min, titrate by 0.02 mcg/min q5 min
      - Dose range: 0.05-0.5 mcg/kg/min; Onset: 1-2 min; Duration: 1-2 min
      - No true max, but consider using additional agents if patient is unresponsive to higher doses.
    - Epinephrine *(second choice)*
      - Infusion: 0.05 mcg/kg/min IV, titrate by 0.02-0.05 mcg/kg/min q15 min
      - Dose range: 0.5 mcg/kg/min; Onset: 1-2 min; Duration: 5-10 min
      - No true max, but consider using additional agents if patient is unresponsive to higher doses.
  - Consider vasopressin 0.03 units/min IV as an alternative to epinephrine in a patient not responding to NE, **OR** in addition to NE with the anticipation of weaning NE dose.
  - Consider phenylephrine or dopamine as third-line therapies.
- **Inotropes: If persistent shock/low ScvO$_2$/or low cardiac index (CI)**
  - Goal CI: 2.6-4.2
  - Dobutamine
    - Infusion: 2.5 mcg/kg/min IV, titrate by 2.5 mcg/kg/min q10 min
    - Max: 20 mcg/kg/min; Onset: 1-2 min; Duration: 10 min
- **Steroids (glucocorticoids):** consider in septic shock refractory to vasopressors.
  - Hydrocortisone
    - Initial dose: 100 mg IV once, **THEN** 200 mg divided q24 hrs
    - Infusion: 200 mg IV given over 24 hrs to minimize both glucose and sodium disturbance
  - ACTH stimulation test is NOT needed.

Source control/antimicrobials

- Mortality benefit when appropriate antibiotics are started **as soon as possible**, with a goal of ≤1 hour of presentation in patients with severe sepsis/septic shock (best practice recommendation); obtain blood cultures x2 prior to initiation if possible.
- **Consider** infection history and local antibiogram data; avoid antibiotics used recently (pathogen is likely to be resistant).
- Empiric antibiotic coverage (dosing based on source). Choose one of the following:
    - Ceftriaxone: 1-2 g IV (2 g if a CNS source is suspected)
    - Piperacillin-tazobactam: 4.5 g IV
    - Cefepime: 1-2 g IV (2 g if patient has neutropenic fever or a CNS source)
    - Doripenem: 500 mg IV
    - Meropenem: 500-1000 mg IV
- **PLUS** vancomycin: 25-30 mg/kg IV (based on actual body weight)
    - Max dose: 2 g IV
- **Consider:** tobramycin/gentamicin: 5-7 mg/kg IV (actual body weight unless obese), **OR** ciprofloxacin: 400 mg IV, as second agent for gram-negative coverage.
- Resistant organisms
    - Atypical pneumonia: azithromycin, 500 mg IV, **OR** doxycycline, 100 mg IV
    - Vancomycin-resistant enterococcus: linezolid, 600 mg IV
    - Multi-drug resistant (MDR) *Pseudomonas* or MDR *Acinetobacter* or MDR *Klebsiella* infections: **ADD** colistimethate, 5 mg/kg (IBW) x1, instead of tobramycin/gentamicin/ciprofloxacin

Additional therapeutic options and considerations

- Source of infection should be identified as soon as possible (goal, within 6 hrs), with appropriate source control (line removal, abscess drainage, etc.) whenever feasible.
- Mechanical ventilation
    - Consider early intubation to decrease metabolic demand.
    - Low tidal volume ventilation (6 mL of tidal volume/kg of predicted body weight)
    - Measure serial plateau pressures with a goal of <30 cm H_2O.
- Check glucose values and treat hyperglycemia.
    - Titrate insulin to a goal of serum glucose <180 mg/dL.
- For antibiotic susceptibilities, consider using local antibiogram, as regional resistance patterns may affect treatment choices.

PEARLS

→ Aggressive fluid resuscitation and early appropriate antibiotic administration are the only treatments with mortality benefit.

→ Patients on vasopressors should have an arterial catheter as soon as possible for accurate BP monitoring.

For any patients with possible toxic exposures or ingestions, consult the **Poison Control** hotline. The national phone number is
1-800-222-1222

ACETAMINOPHEN OVERDOSE

Indications

- Acute ingestions with APAP levels >Rumack-Matthew nomogram *(Table 5)* treatment line.
- Elevated AST and/or INR in ingestions with unknown time window and [APAP] below treatment line.
- History suggesting chronic toxicity with either elevated AST and/or INR or detectable [APAP]. Treat empirically if >150 mg/kg ingestion and [APAP] cannot be obtained within 8 hrs after ingestion.
- *Do not* treat if:
  - Reliable time window is established and [APAP] is below treatment line.
  - Suspected ingestion is >4 hrs ago with undetected APAP level and normal AST.

Treatment

- N-acetylcysteine (NAC): PO and IV routes offer equal protection if given <8 hrs after ingestion.
  - IV NAC: preferable in hepatic failure, pregnancy, or inability to tolerate PO NAC.
    - 21-hr protocol (common)
      - Loading dose: 150 mg/kg over 60 min
      - Second dose: 50 mg/kg/hr for over 4 hrs
      - Third dose: 100 mg/kg/hr for over 16 hrs
    - At end of 21-hour protocol if, it is safe to discontinue NAC therapy if: [APAP] not detectable and AST <1000 or with two down trending values, INR <2, and serum creatinine at baseline. If [APAP] elevated or AST rising or >1000 or evidence significant liver injury, continue NAC at a rate of at least 6.25 mg/kg/hr in consultation with poison center. 6.25 mg/kg/hr is 100 mg/kg over 16 hrs or 150 mg/kg over 24 hrs.
    - Risk of anaphylactoid reaction (up to 20%), especially during loading dose. Give IV NAC in monitored setting. If reaction occurs, hold NAC and give diphenhydramine 25-50 mg IV+/- epinephrine if life-threatening. Consider restarting NAC therapy at half the initial infusion rate or consider PO antidotal therapy.
    - Special dosing: IV dilution required for children <40 kg, max dose obesity 100 kg
  - PO NAC: high incidence of nausea/vomiting; avoid if aspiration risk; use IV NAC over PO unless clear contraindication (active bronchospasm) or not available.
    - 72-hr protocol
      - Loading dose: 140 mg/kg
      - Maintenance doses: 70 mg/kg q4 hrs
      - If vomiting occurs within 1 hr following a given dose, the dose should be repeated.
    - May discontinue therapy if [APAP] is negative, creatinine is at baseline, INR <2, and at least two consecutive AST/ALT measurements are downtrending.
    - To minimize vomiting, dilute in cola soft drink with ice, serve in a covered cup with straw, and administer IV antiemetics.

Additional therapeutic options and considerations

- Activated charcoal (AC): 1 g/kg or 10:1 ratio of AC to APAP
    - No demonstrated benefit if given >2 hrs after APAP ingestion.
    - Contraindicated if there is a concern for aspiration, GI obstruction, or perforations.
- Predictors of fulminant liver failure
    - Serum phosphate level >3 mg/dl measured at 48 to 92 hrs
    - Lactate >3.5 mmol/L after early fluid resuscitation
    - *Modified King's College Hospital Criteria.* List for transplant if:
        - pH is <7.3 or lactate is >3 mmol/L after adequate fluid resuscitation
        - *OR* PT>100 sec, creatinine is >3.3 mg/dl, and there is grade 3 or 4 encephalopathy

Table 5: Matthew-Romack Nomogram

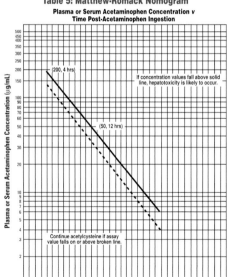

Plasma or Serum Acetaminophen Concentration v Time Post-Acetaminophen Ingestion

Courtesy of www.NIH.gov

→ Consider [APAP] measurement in all patients with intentional overdose, even if no history of acetaminophen ingestion.

→ Contact your poison center and regional transplant center early for all patients you suspect to have impending liver failure.

→ The loading dose of IV NAC must be administered in a monitored unit due to risk of anaphylactoid reaction. Subsequent doses can be administered in a non-monitored unit if patient condition is appropriate.

→ Hold vitamin K and blood products unless significant bleeding is present. INR is a prognostic indicator and important to leave unaffected if patient is not bleeding.

ALCOHOL WITHDRAWAL

Early, uncomplicated withdrawal
- Typically occurs 6-24 hrs after last alcohol ingestion.
- Sx: headache, GI symptoms, diaphoresis, tremulousness, anxiety

Alcoholic hallucinosis
- Can occur while intoxicated, up to 2-3 days after last alcohol ingestion.
- Sx: hallucinations, usually visual; typically normal vital signs

Alcohol withdrawal seizures
- Typically occurs 6-48 hrs after last alcohol ingestion; can occur up to 5 days later.
- Sx: generalized tonic-clonic seizures, status epilepticus very rare

Delirium tremens
- Typically occurs 48 hrs to 1 wk after last alcohol ingestion.
- Sx: confusion, agitation, visual hallucinations, autonomic instability

Treatment

- Symptom-triggered treatment should be basis for therapy, including choice of medication, route (PO, IV, IM) and dose.
- Frequently reassess status and titrate to effect. Indications for repeat dosing: tremor, tachycardia, diaphoresis, agitation, confusion, hallucinations.
- Benzodiazepines
  - Mild-moderate symptoms: chlordiazepoxide: initial dose 25 mg PO, repeat dosing up to 100 mg PO every 6 hrs for 1 day, followed by taper
  - Moderate to severse symptoms:
    - Initial dose: 1-2 mg IV or IM
    - Repeat dosing: titrate to effect, repeat every 10-15 min
  - Diazepam
    - Initial dose: 5-10 mg IV or PO
    - Repeat dosing: titrate up to max of 20 mg IV every 10-15 min

Additional therapeutic options and considerations

- Phenobarbital: 130 mg IV, repeat after 15 min
- Propofol: infusion: 25-200 mcg/kg/min
- Centrally acting alpha-2 agonists
  Clonidine (in uncomplicated withdrawal): initial dose 01.-0.2 mg PO every 8 hrs
  Dexmedetomidine (in severe withdrawal): loading dose: 1 mcg/kg IV over 10 min
  Infusion: 0.2-0.7 mcg/kg/hr

PEARLS

→ Place patient in quiet, protective environment.
→ Use clinical scoring systems such as CIWA (Clinical Institute Withdrawal Assessment) for symptom-triggered therapy.
→ Replete nutritional and electrolyte deficiencies; "banana bags" provide no benefit unless specific deficiencies are noted.
→ Consider underlying condition, especially in refractory cases or persistent tachycardia without agitation.

ANTICHOLINERGIC TOXICITY

Treatment

Cardiac toxicity – wide-complex tachydysrhythmias (i.e., QRS interval >100 msec)
- Sodium bicarbonate
  - Initial dose: 1-2 mEq/kg IV push (usually 50-100 mEq)
  - Infusion: 150 mEq (3 amps) of $NaHCO_3$ in 1L of D_5W at 150-200 cc/hr

Neurotoxicity/central symptoms – agitation, seizures, delirium/hallucinations
- Physostigmine (Antilirium)
  - Initial dose: 1-2 mg (0.02 mg/kg) SLOW IV push over 5 min
    - Have Atropine available in case of precipitating cholinergic crisis ("DUMBELS" – diarrhea, urination, miosis, bronchorrhea/ bronchospasm, emesis, lacrimation, sweating/seizures).
    - Atropine dose: start with half of physostigmine dose administered and titrate to clinical effect.
  - Absolute contraindications: QRS or QT interval prolongation on EKG (reported deaths from asystole when given for TCA overdose with EKG changes), reactive airway disease, epilepsy, or bowel obstruction.
  - Relative contraindications: Reactive airway disease, epilepsy, or bowel obstruction.
  - More effective for delirium and agitation than benzodiazepines.
  - Repeat dosing: q10 min if adequate response is not achieved.
- Benzodiazepines
  - Diazepam: 5-10 mg IV; repeat q5 min as necessary to control symptoms
  - Lorazepam: 1-2 mg IV; repeat q5 min as necessary to control symptoms
  - More effective for seizures than physostigmine.

PEARLS

→ Substances with anticholinergic properties: tricyclic antidepressants, neuroleptics, antihistamines, antiparkinsonian drugs, ophthalmic drugs, and antispasmodics.

→ Clinical diagnosis: red as a beet (flushed skin), dry as a bone (dry skin), hot as a hare (hyperthermia), blind as a bat (nonreactive, dilated pupils), mad as a hatter (hallucinations, delirium), full as a flask (urinary retention), tachycardia (earliest, most reliable), decreased/absent bowel sounds.

→ Physostigmine is indicated if both peripheral and moderate central anticholinergic toxicity are present (mod-severe agitation and delirium).

→ *Sympathomimetic* poisoning may present similarly, but can be differentiated by the presence of diaphoresis and reactive dilated pupils.

→ Neostigmine does not cross the blood-brain-barrier and is not effective at reversing central anticholinergic effect.

BETA-BLOCKER OVERDOSE
Cardiogenic Shock

GI decontamination
- Activated charcoal: 1 g/kg PO (usual dose: 50-100 g)
- Gastric lavage if early presentation (within 1 hr after ingestion)
- *PLUS* whole bowel irrigation for sustained-release preparations
  - Polyethylene glycol electrolyte solution (PEG-3350) via NG *OR* OG tube at 1-2 L/hr until rectal effluent is clear

Pharmacologic therapy
- Normal saline, 0.9% IV bolus, 20 mL/kg (1-2 L in adults); watch for signs of fluid overload/pulmonary edema; may repeat as tolerated.
- Glucagon (be prepared for vomiting)
  - Bolus: 3-5 mg IV (50-150 mcg/kg) over 3-5 min; re-dose 5-10 mg if no effect
  - Infusion: Start maintenance infusion at response dose (3-10 mg/hr), titrate as needed
- Atropine: 0.5-1 mg IV q3-5 min; max, 3 mg total
- *High-dose insulin euglycemia (HIE) therapy*
  - Regular insulin
    - Initial dose: 0.5-1 unit/kg IV with 0.5-1 gm/kg of dextrose IV bolus (1 amp of D_{50} is 25 gms of dextrose)
    - Infusion: 1-10 units/kg/hr IV, start at 1 unit/kg/hr, titrate as needed
    - *PLUS* continuous dextrose infusion at 0.5 g/kg/hr
  - Maintain serum glucose 100-250 mg/dL; recheck glucose q30-60 min.
  - Monitor potassium levels every 60 min and supplement for K^+<3.5 mEq/dL.
- *Consider*
  - Calcium: Treat possible co-ingestion of calcium-channel blocker; may also have small inotropic benefit in isolated β-blocker overdose.
    - Calcium chloride: 1 gm (10% solution) IV via central line (up to 3x)
    - Calcium gluconate: 3 gm (10% solution) by peripheral IV (up to 3x)

- *Intravenous lipid emulsion (ILE) 20%*
  - Dose: 1.5 mL/kg IV bolus (usually 100 mL) over 2-3 min
  - May repeat dose if patient is persistently unstable.
  - If successful, start continuous infusion of ILE 20% 15 mL/kg IV over 60 min.

Blood pressure management
- *Vasopressors and inotropes*
  - Epinephrine, norepinephrine, isoproterenol, or dopamine may be used.
  - May require significantly higher doses than standard infusion; titrate infusion rapidly to effect.
  - Epinephrine 0.05-0.5 mcg/kg/min IV, dopamine 5-20 mcg/kg/min IV, norepinephrine 0.05-0.5 mcg/kg/min IV
  - Consider vasopressin (0.01-0.04 units/min IV) or methylene blue (1-2 mk/kg IV bolus over 20 min followed by continuous IV infusion) in cases of hypotension secondary to vasodilation not responsive to alpha-agonists.

Additional therapeutic options and considerations
- Transcutaneous or transvenous pacemaker
- Phosphodiesterase inhibitors – to treat ventricular dysfunction causing cardiogenic shock
  - Inamrinone, milrinone, enoximone – use standard CHF dosing.
  - Milrinone: load 50 mcg/kg IV over 10 min **THEN** infuse at 0.375 mcg/kg/min IV
- Hemodialysis – nadolol, sotalol, acebutolol, and atenolol can be removed by dialysis.
- Intra-aortic balloon pump
- Extracorporeal membrane oxygenate (ECMO)

PEARLS
→ Patients may present with conduction delays, hypoglycemia (more common in children) or euglycemia, and altered mental status/coma.
→ When using glucagon, give an antiemetic (e.g., ondansetron, 4 mg IV), as it often causes vomiting.
→ Propanolol may cause seizures and QRS interval prolongation and other lipid-soluble β-blockers may cause seizures; treat with benzodiazepines and sodium bicarbonate, respectively.
→ Despite the high doses of insulin that HIE therapy utilizes, respectively lower doses of dextrose are needed to maintain euglycemia as the insulin receptors become saturated in HIE therapy.
→ Consider intiating ECMO early in patients with severe refractory shock or cardiac arrest; ECMO can maintain cardiac output and vital organ perfusion while allowing time for drug redistribution, metabolism, and clearance.

CALCIUM-CHANNEL BLOCKER OVERDOSE
Cardiogenic Shock

GI decontamination
- Activated charcoal: 1 g/kg PO (usual dose: 50-100 g)
- Gastric lavage if early presentation (within 1 hr after ingestion)
- **PLUS** whole bowel irrigation for sustained-release preparations
  - Polyethylene glycol electrolyte solution (PEG-3350) via NG **OR** OG tube at 1-2 L/hr until rectal effluent is clear

Blood pressure management
- Norepinephrine
  - Infusion: 0.05 mcg/kg/min IV, titrate by 0.02 mcg/kg/min q5 min
  - Dose range: 0.05-0.5 mcg/kg/min; Onset: 1-2 min; Duration: 1-2 min
  - No true max, but consider using additional agents if patient is unresponsive to higher doses.

Pharmacologic therapy
- Calcium
  - Initial dose: 13-25 mEq (10-20 mL 10% CaCl by central line **OR** 30-60 mL calcium gluconate by PIV)
  - Infusion: 0.5 mEq/kg/hr **OR** repeat boluses q15-20 min x 3-4 doses
  - Note: 1 g of calcium chloride contains 13.4 mEq of Ca^{2+}; 1 g of calcium gluconate contains 4.3 mEq.
- **High-dose insulin euglycemia (HIE) therapy**
  - Regular insulin
    - Initial dose: 1 unit/kg IV with 1-2 amps of D50 IV bolus
    - Infusion: 1-10 units/kg/hr IV
    - **PLUS** continuous dextrose infusion at 0.5 g/kg/hr, hold for FSG >400 mg/dL
  - Maintain serum glucose 100-250 mg/dL; recheck glucose q30-60 min. Hold bolus for glucose >400 mg/dl.
  - Monitor potassium levels every 60 min and supplement for K^+<3.0 mEq/dL.
- Glucagon (be prepared for vomiting)
  - Initial dose: 3-5 mg IV over 3-5 min, re-dose in 5-10 min if no effect
  - Infusion: 3-10 mg/hr or maintenance at response dose
- Atropine: 0.5-1 mg IV q3-5 min; max: 3 mg total

Additional therapeutic options and considerations
- Intravenous lipid emulsion (ILE) 20%
  - Dose: 1.5 mL/kg IV bolus (usually 100 mL) over 2-3 min
  - May repeat dose if patient is persistently unstable.
  - If successful, start continuous infusion of ILE 20% 15 mL/kg IV over 60 min.

PEARLS

→ CCB overdose is distinguished from BB overdose by the presence of hyperglycemia.
→ Consider CCB toxicity in patients with refractory hypotension, bradycardia, hyperglycemia.
→ Treat all patients suspected of CCB overdose, even if they are asymptomatic; they can decompensate quickly!
→ Symptom onset may be delayed with ingestion of sustained-release formulations.
→ If patient requires pressors, also think about ECMO, intra-aortic balloon pump, or pacemaker.

CHOLINERGIC CRISIS

Indication
- Excess acetylcholine leads to stimulation of both muscarinic and nicotinic receptors.
- *Muscarinic receptor stimulation*
  - **S**alivation, **L**acrimation, **U**rination, **D**efecation, **G**astric **E**mesis, **B**ronchospasm, **B**ronchorrhea, and **B**radycardia (SLUDGE + Killer B's)
- Nicotinic receptor stimulation
  - Fasciculations, muscle weakness, and paralysis
- CNS effects
  - Ataxia, confusion, coma, respiratory depression
- Cardiovascular effects
  - Bradycardia, heart block, QTc prolongation, Torsades de pointes

Treatment
- Decontamination
  - In cases of topical organophosphate exposure, removal of patient clothing and aggressive irrigation of skin is required.
- Activated charcoal: only for ingestion that occurred 1 hour prior to presentation
  - Single dose of 1 g/kg (max 50 g)
- Atropine (muscarinic antagonist)
  - *Adults*
    - Initial dose: 1-4 mg IV *OR* 2-6 mg IM q5-10 min
    - Typically double dose every 5 min until resolution of bronchorrhea and bronchospasm.
  - *Children*
    - Initial dose: 0.05 mg/kg IV *OR* 1 to 2 mg IM q5-10 min
    - Typically double dose every 5 min until resolution of bronchorrhea and bronchospasm.
  - Infusion: Start at 10-20% of total initial loading dose required for control of bronchorrhea and bronchospasm; titrate by 0.02 mg/kg/hr q10 min if frequent dosing is required.
  - Incremental dosing followed by continuous infusion may improve outcomes.

- Pralidoxime (2-PAM) (oximes reactivate inhibited AChEase before receptor aging)
  - *Adults*
    - Loading dose: 1-2 g IV over 30 min; may repeat after 1 hr
    - Maintenance dose: 1-2 g IV q10-12 hrs for 48 hrs **OR**
    - Loading dose: 20 mg/kg (max, 2 gm) IV bolus over 30 min **THEN**
    - Infusion: 8-10 mg/kg/hr (max, 650 mg/hr) IV
  - *Children*
    - Loading dose: 30 mg/kg IV (max: 2 g) over 30 min; may repeat after 1 hr
    - Maintenance: 30 mg/kg IV (max: 2 g) q10-12 hrs for 48 hrs
- Benzodiazepines for cholinergic-induced seizure treatment
  - Diazepam 5-10 mg IV (children 0.05-0.3 mg/kg IV)
  - Lorazepam 2-4 mg IV (children 0.05-0.1 mg/kg IV)
  - Midazolam 5-10 mg IV (children 0.15-0.2 mg/kg IV)

PEARLS

→ Tachycardia and mydriasis are not indications to stop atropine therapy, although HR >120 may indicate sufficient atropinization.

→ Intermediate syndrome presents 24 to 96 hours after exposure with neck flexion weakness, respiratory insufficiency, decreased deep tendon reflexes, and proximal muscle weakness. Thought to be caused by lipophilic organophosphate exposures that were inadequately treated with oximes.

→ Poisoning of acetylcholinesterase prolongs action of succinycholine. Consider rocuronium if paralytic needed.

→ Consider admission for cutaneous exposures, as lipophilic pesticides may cause delayed onset of symptoms.

→ Do not administer 2-PAM without atropine due to transient oxime-induced AChEase inhibition.

→ Hundreds of milligrams of atropine may be required over course of treatment.

CYANIDE TOXICITY

Introduction
- May occur due to smoke inhalation injuries, chemical incidents, intentional exposures.
- Requires decontamination and supportive care.
- Symptomatic patients (delirium, cardiovascular instability) should receive additional treatments below.
- Consider empiric antidotal treatment when exposure is highly suspected.

Treatment
- **Option 1: Cyanokit**
  - Hydroxocobalamin
    - Initial dose: 70 mg/kg (max 5 g) IV over 15 min
    - Second dose can be given if patient is persistently symptomatic.
- **Option 2**
  - Amyl nitrite
    - Give until IV access is established.
    - Initial dose: 1 crushed ample inhaled over 1 min
    - Secondary dosing: repeat every 1 min for 5 min
  - Sodium nitrite
    - Initial dose: 300 mg IV (10 mL)
    - Repeat 150 mg IV if symptoms return.
  - Sodium thiosulfate
    - Initial dose: 12.5 gm IV (50 mL)
    - Repeat 6.25 gm IV if symptoms return.

Additional therapeutic options and considerations
- Treat seizures with benzodiazepines (e.g., lorazepam at standard doses).
- Consider early GI decontamination for oral ingestion if patient has normal mentation.
  - Activated charcoal: 50 g PO once
  - Orogastric lavage if within 60 min after ingestion

PEARLS
→ Always suspect cyanide poisoning in fire victims.
→ May see hyperoxia on VBG due to decreased oxygen utilization by tissues (a narrow arterial-venous oxygen difference).
→ Avoid amyl nitrite and use sodium nitrite with caution in patients with concurrent carbon monoxide poisoning, as methemoglobinemia could be lethal in these patients.
→ Cyanide levels are of no utility in the acute setting.
→ In patients with suspected cyanide poisoning, a lactate level >8 mmol/L correlates with high cyanide levels.
→ Consider adding sodium thiosulfate to hydroxocobalamin therapy.

DIGOXIN TOXICITY
Cardiogenic Shock

Indications for digoxin-specific fab (DSFab)
- Hyperkalemia >5 mEq/L in setting of acute poisoning
- Life-threatening arrhythmias, regardless of digoxin concentration
- Hemodynamic instability
- Digoxin level >10 mcg/mL at least 6 hrs after ingestion
- Lethal dose of digoxin: adults >10 mg; children >4 mg
- Chronic digoxin toxicity is associated with significant GI symptoms or altered mental status.

Treatment
- Initial dose of DSFab
    - Always give half the dose of DSFab over the first 15-20 min.
        - If level or quantity is *unknown*:
            - Dose: 10-20 vials IV
        - If amount of ingestion is *known:*
            - No. of vials = mg ingested/0.5 (mg/vial) x 80%
        - If digoxin level is known:
            - No. of vials = digoxin concentration (mcg/mL) x wt (kg)/100
- Repeat dose of DSFab in 60 min if patient does not improve.
- Give 6 vials for chronic toxicity without a known acute ingestion.

Additional therapeutic options and considerations
- Lidocaine can be used for refractory ventricular dysrhythmias.
    - Loading dose: 1-1.5 mg/kg IV, repeat 0.5-0.75 mg/kg IV q 5-10 min
    - Infusion: 1-4 mg/min IV
    - Max: 300 mg total dose in 1 hr
- Atropine and/or cardiac pacing for symptomatic bradycardia
- Dialysis will not remove digoxin, but may be used to treat digoxin-induced hyperkalemia.
- Magnesium sulfate 2 gm IV over 20 min

PEARLS
→ Use caution if administering calcium for hyperkalemia secondary to digoxin poisoning.
→ Notable arrhythmias include: bidirectional ventricular tachycardia, PVCs, SVT with slow ventricular response.
→ Anticipate hyperkalemia with acute digoxin overdoses.
→ Anticipate hypokalemia with treatment, usually within 4 hrs.
→ 3% of patients will get rebound digoxin toxicity after FAB administration.
→ 40 mg of DSFab neutralizes 0.6 mg of digoxin.
→ After DSFab is administered, total serum digoxin concentrations are no longer useful.

HYDROFLUORIC ACID TOXICITY

An inorganic acid used for glass etching, metal cleaning, and removing rust

Decontamination and supportive care

Clothing removal, copious water irrigation, continuous cardiac monitoring, prepare for possible intubation in inhalation burns.

Cutaneous burns

- *Topical* calcium gluconate 2.5% gel (proprietary gel)
  - To make gel, dissolve 10% Ca^{2+} gluconate in water-soluble lubricant in a 1:3 ratio.
  - For a hand burn, fill glove with gel and place hand inside.
- *Intradermal* calcium gluconate
  - Dose: 0.5 mL of a 5% solution (25-gauge needle or smaller)
    - To make solution, dilute 10% Ca^{2+} gluconate solution with NS in a 1:1 ratio.
    - Calcium chloride is contraindicated due to high risk of local tissue damage.
    - Infiltration not recommended for large surface areas or fingertips, as this may cause precipitation of calcium fluoride and fluorapetite in soft tissue.
  - Dose: 10-15 mL of a 10% solution
    - Mix 10-15 mL of a 10% Ca^{2+} gluconate solution with 4,000 units of heparin and dilute in 20-40 mL of a 5% dextrose solution.
    - Bier ischemic arm-block technique: inflate BP cuff for 20-25 min.
- *Intra-arterial* calcium gluconate
  - Dose: Mix 10-15 mL of a 10% solution in 40 mL of D_5W or lactated Ringer's solution.
  - Infuse over 3-4 hrs via arterial line placement proximal to lesion.

Ocular burns (recommend ophthalmology consult)

- Calcium gluconate (1%) ***irrigation*** for pain following 5 min of water irrigation
  - To make solution, dilute 10% Ca^{2+} gluconate solution with normal saline in 1:10 ratio. *(Do not use undiluted solution.)*

Inhalation burns (may be result of topical exposure to a highly concentrated solution)

- Calcium gluconate: 4 mL of a 2.5% solution ***nebulized*** with 100% oxygen

Oral ingestion

- Calcium chloride: 300 mL of a 10% solution via ***gastric lavage*** (within 60 min after ingestion)

Systemic toxicity

- Calcium gluconate 10% 0.2-0.4 mL/kg IV (repeat liberally)
- Calcium chloride 10% 0.1-0.2 mL/kg IV (central line is preferred)
- Consider magnesium replacement (4 g IV over 20 min)

→ HF exposure should be considered in all patients with potential exposure in whom pain is out of proportion to the exam findings.
→ Fluoride ions complex with calcium and magnesium → hypocalcemia and hypomagnesemia → QTc prolongation and cardiotoxicity → arrhythmias (#1 cause of death with HF burns). Therefore, even very small BSA burns with HF can be potentially life-threatening.
→ With any evidence of hypocalcemia or hyperkalemia, immediately administer 10% calcium gluconate IV.
→ Oral and inhalation exposures should be considered potentially life-threatening.

OPIOID OVERDOSE

Indication
Treatment goal: to reverse *respiratory* depression not CNS depression.

Treatment
- **Respiratory:** hypoventilation (bradypnea or hypopnea)
  - Naloxone
    - Initial dose: 0.04 mg IV bolus; if no response increase to 0.4 mg IV bolus.
    - Titrate cautiously with goal of reversing respiratory depression up to a max 10 mg; lack of response suggests an alternate (or additional) diagnosis.
    - Infusion: 2/3 of the total naloxone bolus dose that resulted in reversal of respiratory depression IV per hour and titrate to effect.
    - Monitor for signs of acute lung injury.
- **Cardiovascular**
  - Hypotension: Treatment is supportive.
  - Bradycardia: Treatment is supportive.

PEARLS
→ The duration of naloxone's effect is often shorter than that of the opioid being reversed. Monitor for symptom recurrence, which may necessitate a continuous naloxone infusion.
→ Administering naloxone to a chronic opioid user who is under the influence of other CNS depressants (e.g., alcohol, benzodiazepines, etc.) may result in a withdrawing (vomiting) patient with a depressed level of consciousness and unprotected airway.
→ QTc prolongation and Torsades de pointes may occur in patients using methadone.
→ Naloxone is well-absorbed by all parenteral routes of administration, including the intramuscular, intranasal, and inhalational (nebulized) routes.

ORAL ANTIHYPERGLYCEMIC AGENT OVERDOSE

Mechanism	Class	Common Drug Names	Side Effects
Table 6: Common Oral Antihyperglycemic Agents and Effects			
"Sensitizers": ↑ sensitivity to insulin	Biguanides	metformin, phenformin	**Lactic acidosis**, diarrhea, B_{12} deficiency
	Thiazolidinediones	rosiglitazone, pioglitazone	Hepatotoxicity, CHF (questionable)
"Secretagogues:" ↑ production of insulin by acting on pancreas; *cause hypoglycemia*	Meglitinides	repaglinide, nateglinide	**Hypoglycemia**, short-acting (<4hrs)
	Sulfonylureas	chlorpropamide glipizide, glyburide, glimepiride, gliclazide	**Hypoglycemia**, chlorpropamide: SIADH, disulfiram-like reaction
↑ Insulin secretion (glucose dependent) ↓ glucagon	Glucagon-like peptide (GLP-1) analogues	exenitide, liraglutide	GI: belching, indigestion. pancreatitis (exenitide), thyroid CA (liraglutide).
DPP-4 inhibitors: stop GLP-1 degradation, ↑insulin, ↓ glucagon	Gliptins	sitagliptin (Januvia), vildagliptin, saxagliptin	Nasopharyngitis (cold-like symptoms), skin lesions
Carbohydrate digestion antagonists	α-Glucosidase inhibitors	acarbose, miglitol, voglibose	Abdominal cramping, diarrhea
SGLT-2 inhibitors: block Na-gluc co-transporter 2	Glycosurics	canagliflozin (Invokana), dapagliflozin	Orthostasis, UTIs, mycotic infxns (balanitis, vaginitis), electrolyte disorder (↑K+)

Secretagogues

Hypoglycemic symptoms – two subdivisions

- *Neuroglycopenia:* coma, delirium, seizure, focal neuro deficits
- *Catecholamine-related:* diaphoresis, shaking, anxiety (blunted by β-blockers!)
- Specific medications are listed in *Table 6*.

Treatment

GI decontamination

- Consider for oral secretagogue overdose (i.e., sulfonylureas and meglitinides).
- Activated charcoal: <2 hrs after ingestion to decrease absorption
  - Use caution if patient has AMS or risk of aspiration.
  - Dose: 50-100 g PO
- Avoid ipecac, gastric lavage, or whole bowel irrigation.

Pharmacologic management

- Restore euglycemia.
  - Key point: Give supplemental glucose *only* if hypoglycemia is present.
  - If hypoglycemia *is* present (glucose <60 mg/dL *OR* <90 mg/dL with AMS)
    - Dextrose: 0.5 to 1 g/kg IV
      - Adults: 1 amp of D_{50} IV bolus
      - Toddlers/children: 2 mL/kg D_{25} IV
      - Infants: 5 mL/kg D_{10} IV
    - Feed patient a complex carbohydrate-rich meal to maintain euglycemia.
  - Refractory hypoglycemia – glucose infusion
    - Infusion: Start at weight-appropriate maintenance and titrate to euglycemia.
    - Peripheral IV: $D_{10}W$
    - Central line: $D_{25}W$ (requires central line, sclerosing to PIVs)
- Decrease insulin release.
  - Octreotide: *should be given if patient does not respond to initial glucose bolus or requires multiple glucose boluses.*
    - Dose: 1-2 mcg/kg IV *OR* SQ q8 hrs x 24 hrs
- Disposition
  - Admit any pediatric patient with a possible sulfonylurea ingestion for 24 hrs of observation.
  - Observe any adult sulfonylurea overdose for 12 hrs of serial blood glucose monitoring and admit if any hypoglycemic episodes.

Biguanides

Lactic acidosis

- Incidental in therapeutic use, but life-threatening in overdose.
  - Associated with 30-50% mortality.
- Severe acidosis leads to hemodynamic instability and mental status depression.

Treatment

Monitoring

- Monitor ABCs.
- Follow serial BMP, lactate, pH q1-2 hrs in large overdoses.

Pharmacologic management — biguanides

- Fluid hydration to optimize renal metformin clearance
- Severe acidosis:
  - pH <7.2 associated with increased mortality
  - Sodium bicarbonate bolus and infusion to correct acidosis

- Hemodialysis (HD):
  - Consider nephrology consultation for pH <7.2, rapidly increasing lactate, decreasing pH, hemodynamic compromise.
  - Corrects acidosis and removes metformin.
  - *Initiate early;* hemodynamic instability may prohibit use.
- Continuous veno-venous hemofiltration (CVVH) if too unstable for HD.
  - Not as effective as HD.

PEARLS

→ Pediatric patients with an oral sulfonylurea overdose should be admitted and observed for at least 24 hrs.

→ $D_{50}W$ is sclerosing to pediatric veins, as is $D_{25}W$ for infants; case reports of seizures and coma.

→ Consider glucagon, 5 mg IM, as temporizing agent if patient is symptomatic and no IV access is available. Less efficacious in children.

→ Consider IO dextrose administration if peripheral access cannot be established.

→ Monitor potassium and phosphate; insulin/glucose can cause profound ↓K and ↓phos.

→ If patient has taken an intentional overdose, check for co-ingestants (APAP, ASA, ECG, UDS).

PIT-VIPER ENVENOMATION

Indication

Envenomation with (1) hemodynamic compromise, (2) significant coagulopathy or thrombocytopenia, (3) neuromuscular toxicity, or (4) progression of swelling

General Management

- Treat pain and anxiety with analgesics (opioids) and anxiolytics (benzodiazepines).
- Address tetanus status.
- Immobilize the extremity in a well-padded splint in near-full extension, and elevate to prevent dependent edema.

Treatment

- CroFab – Crotalidae polyvalent immune Fab
  - Initial dose: depends on severity
    - **Mild:** 4 vials; **Moderate:** 4-6 vials; **Severe:** 8-12 vials
      - Starting dose should be diluted in 250 mL of 0.9% normal saline.
      - Start infusion slowly (25-50 cc/hr) for 10 min and if tolerated, deliver the entire dose in 1 hr.
      - May infuse faster if patient is critically ill.
    - Repeat with an additional 4- to 6-vial doses if control is not achieved with the initial dose. Continue to treat with 4- to 6-vial doses until local manifestations, coagulation tests, and systemic signs are normal.

- After control has been established (swelling is arrested and fibrinogen, prothrombin time, and platelets are showing clear improvement), give 2 vials every 6 hrs for up to 18 hrs. This may not be necessary for many copperhead and cottonmouth bites.

Additional therapeutic options and considerations

- Supportive airway and cardiovascular treatment should be anticipated.
- Place bite injury in elevation and generously use narcotics to alleviate pain.
- Current literature does not endorse the use of fasciotomy. CroFab use has been associated with decreased compartment pressures. Compartment pressures should not be measured routinely.

PEARLS

→ Rattlesnake envenomations are usually worse than cottonmouth/copperhead bites.
→ 25% of bites result in no envenomation; however, at least 8 hrs of observation are needed due to delayed reactions (increased to 24 hrs for children).
→ Possible sequelae include localized pain and edema, hematologic changes (thrombocytopenia, coagulopathies), neurologic toxicity (paresthesias, fasciculations), systemic signs (hypotension, tachycardia).
→ IV Crofab: Hypersensitivity reactions (pruritus, rash, urticaria) are seen in 5.4% of patients.
→ CroFab is contraindicated in patients with known hypersensitivity to papaya/papain unless benefits outweigh risks (caution with anaphylaxis).
→ Avoid: incision and/or suction of wound, ice, NSAIDs, prophylactic antibiotics, steroids (except for allergic reactions), tourniquets, routine use of blood products.

SALICYLATE OVERDOSE

Definition: Toxicity is >150 mg/kg; lethal dose is >500 mg/kg.

Treatment

- **Airway**
    - Key to RSI is to minimize the apneic time as CO_2 retention can acutely worsen the acidosis. Have the most experienced physician intubate, or consider awake intubation.
    - After intubation, set vent to match patient's pre-intubation respiratory rate.
    - If severely acidotic, premedication with 2-4 amps of $NaHCO_3$ may be considered.
- **Charcoal** (1-2 g/kg PO)
    - Consider repeat doses of activated charcoal if there is evidence of ongoing absorption (i.e., salicylate level rising).
    - Serum alkalinization: sodium bicarbonate ($NaHCO_3$) if salicylate level >30 mg/dL
        - Bolus: 1-2 mEq/kg IV push
        - Infusion: 1 liter D5W + 3 amps of $NaHCO_3$ (150 mEq) at 2-3 ml/kg/hr
            - 1 amp of 8.4% $NaHCO_3$ = 50 mL; 1 mL=1 mEq
            - *Do not mix* $NaHCO_3$ with NS, as this will create a hypertonic solution.
        - Goal is blood pH 7.45-7.55; there is no need to measure urinary pH.

- **Fluids and electrolytes** (repeat ABG and electrolytes every 2-3 hours)
    - Serial glucose measurements: for hypoglycemia
    - Monitor potassium: Add 40 mEq of K+ after confirming adequate urine output.
    - Goal urine output is 1-1.5 mL/kg
- **Dialysis indications**
    - Serum salicylate levels
        - Acute poisoning: >90-100 mg/dL (irrelevant of symptoms)
        - Chronic poisoning: >60 mg/dL or any of the symptoms below
    - Non-cardiogenic pulmonary edema (NCPE)
    - Altered mental status or seizures (cerebral edema)
    - Renal failure
    - Severe acidosis or hypotension refractory to supportive treatment

PEARLS

→ Patient's ASA toxicity can present similarly to sepsis, DKA, thyroid storm, and psychiatric agitation.
→ Don't forget about *chronic* poisoning (especially in elderly or psychiatric patients).
→ Don't wait for the levels to come back. Treat immediately!
→ Causes of arrest include severe acidemia and hypo-k.
→ Severe dehydration may occur from vomiting, hyperthermia, and hyperventilation. Give IVF, but watch for noncardiogenic pulmonary edema.
→ Other common salicylates include methyl salicylate (oil of wintergreen, BenGay) and bismuth subsalicylate (Pepto-Bismol).
→ Repeat serum aspirin levels every 2-3 hours until peak concentration is reached, followed by a decrease (half-life in OD is up to 20 hours).

TOXIC ALCOHOL INGESTION

Indications

- Treatment for accidental/intentional ingestions with:
    - Methanol: alcohol odor, found in windshield wiper fluid and gas line antifreeze
    - Ethylene glycol: odorless, sweet tasting, found in radiator antifreeze
    - Isopropanol: aromatic odor, bitter tasting, found in rubbing alcohol

Treatment

- There is NO role for activated charcoal/gastric emptying (unless co-ingestants are suspected).
- **Fomepizole** inhibits alcohol dehydrogenase from producing toxic metabolites.
- Isopropyl alcohol can be toxic, but it is rapidly metabolized to acetone, which mainly causes CNS depression. Fomepizole is not indicated for isopropanol poisoning.
- Indications
    - Suspected ingestion of ethylene glycol or methanol until concentrations are available

- Coma/AMS in patient with unexplained osmolar gap or unexplained anion-gap acidosis with ethanol level <100 mg/dL
- Ethylene glycol or methanol concentrations >20 mg/dL
- Loading dose: 15 mg/kg IV over 30 min
- Maintenance dose: 10 mg/kg IV q12 hrs x 4 doses starting 12 hrs after loading dose
  - If continued beyond the first 4 maintenance doses, must increase back to 15 mg/kg
  - Continue therapy until alcohol levels are confirmed to be <20 mg/dL.
  - Adjust dosing in patients undergoing hemodialysis.
- **Ethanol** (competes for alcohol dehydrogenase, requires central line)
  - Consider only if fomepizole is unavailable.
  - Loading dose: 0.6 g ethanol/kg IV
  - Maintenance infusion: 100 mg/kg/hr, titrate to serum EtOH of 100 mg/dL
    - ICU monitoring is required. Complications include hypotension, hypoglycemia, hyponatremia, pancreatitis, gastritis, and inebriation.
    - Orally administered ethanol also is effective.
- **Hemodialysis**
  - Definitive removal of parent toxic alcohol, metabolites, and correction of acidosis.
  - Ethylene glycol can sometimes be treated with fomepizole alone if kidney function remains intact; methanol usually needs dialysis because its main elimination path is the lungs (slow).
  - Indications for methanol and ethylene glycol ingestions:
    - Refractory metabolic acidosis pH <7.25 or base deficit >15
    - Visual abnormalities
    - Renal insufficiency
    - Deteriorating vital signs
    - Electrolyte abnormalities refractory to conventional therapy
    - Serum methanol or ethylene glycol level >50 mg/dL, unless arterial pH >7.30

PEARLS

→ Isopropanol requires supportive care. Hallmark is osmolar gap WITHOUT anion gap and more inebriation/gastritis than other toxic alcohols.

→ Sodium bicarbonate infusion should be considered in severe metabolic acidosis. Titrate to pH >7.20.

→ Ethylene glycol causes the formation of calcium oxalate crystals, which may be present in the urine.

→ Methanol can lead to blindness via formate retinal injury.

→ High osmolar gap usually is seen early (although neither sensitive nor specific), and high anion gap is seen late.

→ Ethylene glycol can cause elevated lactic acid (usually <5). The glycolate metabolite may cause a false-positive lactate elevation (>5) when measured by some analyzers.

→ Adjunctive thiamine (100 mg IV x 1) and pyridoxine (10-20 mg PO/IV/IM) should be given for ethylene glycol poisoning and folic acid (1 mg PO) for methanol poisoning.

TRICYCLIC ANTIDEPRESSANT (TCA) OVERDOSE

Overdose can lead to blockage of fast sodium channels (arrhythmias, hypotension); antagonism of muscarinic receptors (anticholinergic effects), α1 adrenergic receptors (hypotension), histamine receptors (somnolence, AMS), and GABA receptors (seizures). Commonly prescribed TCAs include amitriptyline, desipramine, nortriptyline, and imipramine.

Treatment

General

- **IMMEDIATE** ECG; fingerstick glucose, acetaminophen and salicylate levels
- Consider early intubation as patients can decompensate quickly with decreased mental status and seizures.
- Benzodiazepines for severe agitation and/or seizures
- Activated charcoal (1 gm/kg)
  - If no risk of aspiration
  - Time since ingestion <2 hours

Cardiotoxicity

- *If QRS interval >100 msec:*
  - Sodium bicarbonate (NaHCO₃)
    - Initial dose: 1-2 mEq/kg IV bolus
    - Repeat bolus until QRS remains <100 msec
    - Infusion: 150 mEq NaHCO₃ in D₅W at 250 cc/hr
      - Monitor electrolytes and pH q1 hr
    - Goal is hemodynamic stability, QRS <100 msec and pH 7.45-7.55
  - Run continuous EKG; QRS interval should narrow within 60 sec of bicarbonate administration.

Hypotension (due to cardiac depression and peripheral vasodilation)

- Initial treatment with bicarbonate therapy and normal saline IVF resuscitation
- Vasopressors → indicated for hypotension refractory to NaHCO₃ and NS
  - Norepinephrine:
    - Infusion: Initiate at 0.02 mcg/kg/min, titrate to MAP >65
  - Epinephrine:
    - Infusion: Initiate at 0.01 mcg/kg/min, titrate to MAP >65
  - Phenylephrine:
    - Infusion: 1-5 mcg/kg/min, titrate to MAP >65
  - Alpha agonists preferred agent given alpha-antagonist effect of TCAs

Seizures (due to GABA receptor inhibition)

- Benzodiazepines are treatment of choice.
  - Midazolam:
    - Initial dose: 5-10 mg IV bolus
  - Lorazepam:
    - Initial dose: 4 mg IV bolus
  - Diazepam:
    - Initial dose: 5-10 mg IV bolus

- For status epilepticus requiring intubation
  - Propofol
  - Phenobarbital

Additional therapeutic options and considerations
- Hypertonic saline 3%: for hypotension refractory to vasopressors
  - Bolus: 100 cc IV, repeat q 10 minutes x 2 doses if needed
- Magnesium: consider for arrhythmia refractory to bicarbonate.
- Lidocaine: consider for arrhythmia refractory to sodium bicarbonate.
  - Initial dose: 1-1.5 mg/kg IV q3-5 min
  - Max dose: 3 mg/kg IV
- IV lipid emulsion (ILE) 20%: for cases refractory to standard therapy with severe hemodynamic instability.
  - Consider strongly while early in course.
  - Initial bolus: 1.5 mL/kg IV bolus over 2-3 min, repeat x1 if unstable
  - If successful, start continuous infusion ILE 20% 15 mL/kg IV over 60 min.

PEARLS
→ TCA levels of little value in the acute setting; the clinical picture dictates the need for treatment.

→ Acute toxic ingestions (>10 mg/kg) usually manifest with severe cardiovascular and CNS effects within 6 hrs, although absorption can be delayed.

→ Classic ECG findings include: sinus tachycardia; right-axis deviation of the terminal 40 msec (positive terminal R wave in lead aVR, and a negative S wave in leads 1 and aVL); and a prolongation of the PR, QRS, and QTc intervals.

→ QRS interval >100 msec portends a 33% risk of seizures; >160 msec, a 50% risk of ventricular dysrhythmias.

→ Class 1A and 1C antidysrhythmics are **contraindicated**; physostigmine to treat anticholinergic effects is **contraindicated**.

→ After 6 hours with no signs or symptoms of toxicity (QRS <100 msec, HR <120, no dysrhythmias, no hypotension, no AMS/seizures, no ↓ bowel sounds) patients can be cleared for psychiatric evaluation.

CARDIOGENIC SHOCK

Differential Diagnosis

- Congenital heart disease (left-sided obstructive lesions)
- Infectious myocarditis
- Arrhythmias
- Congestive heart failure
- Ischemic heart disease
- Cardiomyopathy
- Cardiac tamponade
- Late sepsis
- Drugs (acute and chronic)
- Infiltrative disease (mucopolysaccharidoses, glycogen storage diseases)
- Systemic hypertension

Treatment

- IV fluid resuscitation
  - 0.9% normal saline bolus: 10 mL/kg IV bolus
    - If MAP <65 (dependent on age) after 20 mL/kg, consider inotropic medications.
    - Be judicious, as there is a potential for exacerbation of cardiogenic failure in cardiomyopathy and congenital heart disease.
- *Vasopressors*
  - Dopamine
    - Initial dose: 1-5 mcg/kg/min IV
    - Infusion: 5 mcg/kg/min IV, titrate by 5 mcg/kg/min q10 min
    - Max: 50 mcg/kg/min; Onset: 5 min; Duration: <10 min
      - Has exhibited nonlinear kinetics in peds; may not achieve steady state for approximately 1 hr.
  - Epinephrine
    - Infusion: 0.05 mcg/kg/min IV, titrate by 0.02-0.05 mcg/kg/min q15 min
    - Dose range: 0.05-2 mcg/kg/min; Onset: 1-2 min; Duration: 5-10 min
    - No true max, but consider using additional agents if patient is unresponsive to higher doses.
    - Usual dose range in cardiac patients is 0.03-0.3 mcg/kg/min, after which $\alpha > \beta$ and no longer predominantly inotropic.
    - Beware of peripheral ischemic changes and/or increase in lactate.
  - Norepinephrine $\alpha > \beta$
    - Infusion: 0.05 mcg/kg/min IV, titrate by 0.02 mcg/kg/min q5 min
    - Dose range: 0.05-2 mcg/kg/min; Onset: 1-2 min; Duration: 1-2 min
    - No true max, but consider using additional agents if patient is unresponsive to higher doses.

- **Inotropic agents**
  - Dobutamine
    - Infusion: Initiate at 2.5 mcg/kg/min IV, titrate by 2.5 mcg/kg/min q10 min
    - Max: 20 mcg/kg/min; Onset: 1-2 min; Duration: 10 min
      - β-1 agonist, therefore risk of hypotension and tachycardia
      - Children under 2 years old may have a reduced response.
      - If minimal response, consider epinephrine.
  - Milrinone: phosphodiesterase inhibitor
    - Infusion: 0.375 mcg/kg/min IV, titrate by 0.005 mcg/kg/min q5-10 min
    - Max: 0.75 mcg/kg/min; Onset: 5-15 min
      - Increases contractility and decreases afterload.
      - May cause reflex tachycardia due to peripheral vasodilation.
      - Useful as adjunct to epinephrine; allows higher epinephrine dosing with persistent effect as pure inotrope.
      - Dosing adjustments may be necessary for renal impairment.
- **Prostoglandins**
  - Prostaglandin E1 (Alprostadil)
    - Initial dose: 0.05-0.1 mcg/kg/min
    - Infusion: 0.01-0.4 mcg/kg/min (reduce rate to lowest effective dosage)
    - Onset: ~15 min-11 hrs (for acyanotic congenital heart disease)
    - Duration: 1-2 hrs
      - Start if suspicion for ductal-dependent lesion in a *normal* neonate to maintain or re-establish patency of the ductus arteriosus.
      - Should be given through an umbilical artery catheter or a large vein.
      - Ductus arteriosus closes by 3rd week of life in the term neonate; may be later in the pre-term neonate.
      - Side effects include apnea and hypotension.

PEARLS

→ Initial presentation may be identical to hypovolemic shock; give IV fluids. If no response or worsening, suspect cardiogenic shock.

→ Obtain a bedside echocardiogram early to help differentiate types of shock.

→ Consider a ductal-dependent lesion if patient is presenting in first 1-2 weeks of life with shock, cyanosis, hepatomegaly, tachypnea, poor feeding, or diaphoresis with feeding.

→ Neonates and infants have limited glycogen stores, which may become rapidly depleted during shock; obtain blood glucose level early and often and add dextrose as needed.

→ Multiple-system organ support may be required, including modalities such as mechanical ventilation, renal dialysis, ventricular assist devices (VAD), or even extracorporeal membrane oxygenation (ECMO).

→ Optimize ionized calcium to maximize cardiac contractility, as infant myocardium is exquisitely sensitive to hypocalcemia.

→ In newborns, if both preductal and postductal oxygen saturations are <95% or if there is a >3% difference between the two, there is a high likelihood of congenital heart disease.

SEPTIC SHOCK
Distributive Shock

Definition
- SIRS: 2 out of 4 of the following, must include temperature:
  - Core temperature >38.5° C or <36° C
  - Tachycardia >2 standard deviations (SD) for age or bradycardia <10th percentile for age
  - Respiratory rate >2 SD for age
  - Age specific ↓ or ↑ WBC count or >10% bandemia
- Septic shock: SIRS with end-organ hypoperfusion in the setting of presumed infection. ≥2 of the following constitute shock:
  - Metabolic acidosis, lactate >4 mmol/L
  - Altered mental status
  - Capillary refill time >5 sec
  - Oliguria <0.5 mL/kg/hr
  - Core: peripheral temperature gap >3°C
- WARM SHOCK (early finding): warm extremities (↓ systemic vascular resistance (SVR) or peripheral vasodilation), bounding pulses (↑ stroke volume, cardiac index, and wide pulse pressure)
- COLD SHOCK (late finding): cool extremities (↑ SVR), prolonged capillary refill time, oliguria

Treatment
- *Fluid resuscitation*
  - 0.9% normal saline boluses of 20 ml/kg to goal of 60 ml/kg in first hour
    - Goal cardiac index (CI=SV x HR/BSA): 3.3-6 L/min/m^2
    - Goal urine output >1 mL/kg/hr
- *Antibiotics* INITIATE EARLY
  - Vary by age, suspected source, and local sensitivities
- *Vasoactive therapy goals:* start within 1st hr in fluid refractory shock; may use peripherally until central access is obtained.
  - Dynamic adjustments to hemodynamic support to maintain CI: vasopressor alone for isolated ↓SVR, vasopressor *PLUS* inotrope for combined ↓ SVR and ↓ CI, *OR* inotrope *PLUS* vasodilator for ↓ CI *PLUS* ↑SVR
  - Dopamine (first-line vasoactive agent)
    - Infusion: 5 mcg/kg/min IV, titrate by 5 mcg/kg/min q10 min
    - Max: 50 mcg/kg/min; Onset: 3-5 min (<6 mos can be insensitive)
- *Fluid-resistant, dopamine-resistant shock: additional vasoactive agent*
  - Norepinephrine for WARM SHOCK (↓ CI and ↓ SVR)
    - Infusion: 0.05 mcg/kg/min IV, titrate by 0.02 mcg/kg/min q5 min
    - Dose range: 0.05-2 mcg/kg/min; Onset: 1-2 min; Duration: 1-2 min
    - No true max, but consider using additional agents if patient is unresponsive to higher doses.

- Epinephrine for COLD SHOCK ($\downarrow$ CI and $\uparrow$ SVR)
    - Infusion: 0.05 mcg/kg/min IV, titrate by 0.02-0.05 mcg/kg/min q15 min
    - Dose range: 0.05-2 mcg/kg/min; Onset: 1-2 min; Duration: 5-10 min
        - No true max, but consider using additional agents if patient is unresponsive to higher doses. Inotropic agents: initiate for $\downarrow$ CI.
- ***Inotropes: Epinephrine-resistant shock: initiate for $\downarrow$ CI and $\uparrow$ SVR***
    - Milrinone: inodilator may $\uparrow$ CI and $\downarrow$ SVR
        - Loading dose: 50 mcg/kg IV over 10-15 min
        - Infusion: 0.375 mcg/kg/min IV, titrate by 0.005 mcg/kg/min q5-10 min
        - Max: 0.75 mcg/kg/min; Onset: 5-15 min; Duration: variable
            - Dosing adjustment required for renal impairment
            - Synergistic effect with B-adrenergic agonists
            - NOTE: long elimination half-life; discontinue at first sign of hypotension
    - Dobutamine: May increase CI in refractory shock.
        - Infusion: 2.5 mcg/kg/min IV, titrate by 2.5 mcg/kg/min q10 min
        - Max: 20-40 mcg/kg/min; Onset: 1-2 min; Duration: 10 min

Additional therapeutic options and considerations

- ***Glucose:*** Children in septic shock have high glucose demands due to limited glycogen stores.
    - Glucose IV bolus *(Rule of 50s)*
        - <1 year of age: 5 mL/kg D_{10}
        - 1-8 years: 2 mL/kg D_{25}
        - >8 years: 1 mL/kg D_{50}
    - Check glucose early and often. Consider maintenance IVF with glucose if needed.
- ***Steroids:*** Use for fluid-refractory and vasopressor-dependent shock, patients on chronic steroids, patients with known or presumed adrenal insufficiency (basal cortisol <18 mcg/dL), or adrenal-pituitary axis failure.
    - Hydrocortisone: 0.5 mg/kg IV q6 hrs
- ***Transfusion:*** Consider if Hgb <10, $ScvO_2$ <70%, or minimal response to IV fluid bolus of 60-80 mL/kg.
    - Packed RBC transfusion: 10-20 cc/kg
- ***Consider ECMO in refractory shock.***

Pearls

→ Children in shock present differently than adults in shock – hypotension is a late sign.
→ Pediatric septic shock is more frequently due to low cardiac output, as opposed to low systemic vascular resistance in adults.
→ Aggressive fluid resuscitation and early initiation of antibiotic therapy are the most critical interventions in septic shock.
→ Dynamic adjustments to hemodynamic support after 60 mL/kg fluid resuscitation in the first hour and dopamine infusion are critical. Choice of additional vasoactive agent depends on findings consistent with cold vs. warm shock.

SEDATION

Indication

The role of sedation in children is the management of pain, anxiety, and control of excessive movement when it could interfere with a diagnosis and/or treatment plan.

- Sedation is commonly warranted in preparation for the following procedures:
  - Abscess incision and drainage
  - Arthrocentesis
  - Bone marrow biopsy
  - Burn debridement
  - CT or MRI
  - Dislocation
  - Foreign body removal
  - Fracture reduction
  - Lumbar puncture
  - Sexual assault exam
  - Suturing/wound care
  - Tube thoracostomy

Table 7: Commonly Used Agents for Pediatric Sedation

Medication	Dose	Route	Interval	Peak Effect	Duration
Analgesia					
Fentanyl	<6 yrs: 0.3-1.5 µg/kg/dose >6 yrs: 1.2 µg/kg/dose	IV (slow push)	q1-2 hrs	15 min	60 min
	1.5-2 µg/kg	Nasal	q15 min	15 min	60 min
Morphine	0.08-0.1 mg/kg/dose	IV	q5-10 min	15-30 min	1-3 hrs
	0.08-0.1 mg/kg/dose	IM	q5-10 min	30-60 min	1-3 hrs
Sedative/Anxiolytic					
Midazolam	6 mos-5 yrs: 0.05-0.1 mg/kg (max: 6 mg); 6-12 yrs: 0.025-0.05 mg/kg (max:10 mg)	IV	q10-15 min	5-10 min	1-4 hrs
	0.25-1 mg/kg/dose (max 20 mg)	PO	once	30 min	1-4 hrs
	0.1-0.15 mg/kg/dose (max 10 mg)	IM	once	10-15 min	1-4 hrs
	0.2-0.5 mg/kg/dose	Nasal	once	10-15 min	1-4 hrs
Diazepam	0.25 mg/kg/dose (max 10 mg)	IV/IM	q15-30 min	15-30 min	60 min
	2-5 yrs: 0.5 mg/kg/dose 6-11 yrs: 0.3 mg/kg/dose >12 yrs: 0.2 mg/kg/dose	Rectal	q15-30 min	15-30 min	60 min
Pentobarbital	1-6 mg/kg/dose (max 100 mg/dose)	IV (slow push)	q1 hr	3-5 min	15-45 min
	2-6 mg/kg/dose (max 100 mg/dose)	IM	q1 hr	10-20 min	1-2 hrs
Sedative/Hypnotic					
Ketamine	Initial: 1-1.5 mg/kg/dose Maintenance: 0.5 mg/kg/dose	IV (slow push) IV	once q10-15 min	1 min	10-15 min
	Initial: 4 mg/kg/dose Maintenance: 2-4 mg/kg/dose	IM IM	once q15-30 min	5-10 min	15-30 min
Propofol	0.5-1 mg/kg/dose	IV (slow push)	q3-5 min	<1 min	1-3 min
	125-150 µg/kg/min	Infusion	continuous	continuous	3-5 min
Nitrous oxide	1:1 oxygen: nitrous oxide	Inhaled	continuous	30-60 min	5 min
Dexmedeto-midine	0.2-0.7 µg/kg/hr	Infusion	continuous	15-25 min	30 min
Chloral hydrate	50-100 mg/kg/dose (max 2 g)	PO	q6 hrs	60 min	5-9 hrs

PEARLS

→ Consider length and pain of procedure when choosing medication and dose.
→ Don't forget topical adjuncts (i.e., transdermal lidocaine, EMLA, LET, LMX).
→ Have reversal agents such as naloxone for opioids and flumazenil for
   benzodiazepine overdose readily available.
   – Naloxone: 0.01 mg/kg IV q 2-3 min
   – Flumazenil: 0.0.1 mg/kg IV (max dose 0.2 mg)
→ If control of oral secretions is critical, consider atropine 0.01-0.02 mg/kg (min 0.1 mg
   to avoid paradoxical bradycardia).
→ Fentanyl can cause respiratory depression – all opioids can. However, chest wall
   rigidity is associated with fentanyl only.
→ Nasal midazolam burns for 30 seconds.

Disclaimer: The following information is extrapolated from case reports and operating room scenarios. No peer-reviewed data exists on outcome studies or maximum dosing when used in an emergency department setting. Caution must be exercised when applying this information to individual clinical scenarios.

Indication: Temporary relief of hypotension

- Peri-intubation hypotension
- Hypotension in procedural sedation
- Bridge to long-term vasopressor use
- Hypotension produced by spinal epidural anesthesia

- **Phenylephrine:** pure α1-agonist causing arterial vasoconstriction
  - Dose: 50-200 mcg IV q2-5 min (0.5-2 mL of 100 mcg/mL phenylephrine) to goal BP
  - Onset: 1 min; Duration: 15-20 min
  - Instructions to create 100 mcg/mL
    - Add 1 mL of 10 mg/mL phenylephrine to 100 mL of normal saline (NS).

- **Epinephrine:** mixed α/β agonist
  Consider when inotropy and vasoconstriction are needed.
  - Dose: 5-20 mcg IV q2-5 min (0.5-2 mL of 10 mcg/mL epinephrine) to desired effect
  - Onset: 1 min; Duration: 5-10 min
  - Instructions to create 10 mcg/mL:
    - Add 1 mL of 100 mcg/mL *OR* 1:10,000 epinephrine to 9 mL of NS.

- **Ephedrine:** mixed α/β agonist
  - Dose: 5-10 mg IV q2-5 min (1-2 mL of 5 mg/mL ephedrine) to desired effect
  - Onset: 2-5 min; Duration: 60 min
  - Instructions to create 5 mg/mL:
    - Add 1 mL of a 50 mg/mL-vial to 9 mL of NS.
  - Rarely used because of longer half-life and cardiac complications.
  - Consider when both inotropic augmentation and vasoconstriction are needed.

Additional therapeutic options and considerations

- Based on use in an operative setting; best results are obtained when systolic blood pressure or heart rate is decreased by >30% from baseline or when systolic blood pressure is <100 mmHg.
- Ephedrine (an indirectly acting sympathomimetic amine) is best reserved for previously healthy patients undergoing procedures expected to yield temporary hypotensive episodes (e.g., spinal anesthesia, procedural sedation).

PEARLS

→ All the medications listed above can be administered through a peripheral IV without fear of complications should extravasation occur.

→ Care must be taken, as phenylephrine — but not ephedrine — decreases cardiac output and brain oxygenation in anesthetized patients and produces a reflex bradycardia.

→ The use of single-dose phenylephrine and ephedrine has shown a decrease in intra-operative nausea and vomiting; therefore, there is a theoretical decrease in aspiration when applied to an emergency setting.

→ The use of single-dose phenylephrine and ephedrine has shown a decrease in intra-operative nausea and vomiting. There is a theoretical decrease in aspiration when applied to an emergency setting.

TARGETED TEMPERATURE MANAGEMENT (TTM)

Indication

- Comatose survivors of cardiac arrest, regardless of initial rhythm.
- "Comatose" is defined as a lack of meaningful response to verbal commands.
- Current guidelines recommend a target temperature of 32-34°C (89.6°F to 93.2°F) for 12 to 24 hrs; recent evidence indicates that 36°C (98.6°F) may be as effective.

Treatment

Induction phase

- Infusion of 4°C crystalloids (LR or NS): 30 mL/kg as bolus; alone or in conjunction with:
    - Ice packs to groin, axillae, head, and neck
    - Cooling blankets
    - Endovascular cooling devices with feedback technology
- Monitor temperature:
    - Esophageal probe placement *(First choice)*
    - Temperature-sensing Foley in non-anuric patients *(Second choice)*
    - Rectal probe *(Third choice)*
    - Pulmonary artery catheter; *if* placed for other indications, can also be used to monitor core temperature
    - **Do not use** axillary, oral, or tympanic measurements.
- If sedation is required or shivering is not controlled, consider the following:
    - Propofol
        - Infusion: 5 mcg/kg/min, titrate by 5-10 mcg/kg/min q5 min PRN
        - Onset: ~30 sec; Duration: 3-10 min
    - Midazolam
        - Loading dose: 0.01-0.05 mg/kg IV; may repeat at 10-15 min PRN
        - Infusion (maintenance): 0.02-0.1 mg/kg/hr; titrate 0.025 mg/kg/hr q2-3 min
        - Onset: 3-5 min; Duration: variable
    - Dexmedetomidine
        - *Consider an alternative agent if the patient is experiencing bradycardia.*
        - Infusion (maintenance): 0.2-0.7 mcg/kg/hr, titrate by 0.1 mcg/kg/hr q15 min
            - Doses up to 1.4 mcg/kg/hr have been reported.
        - Onset: 5-10 min; Peak: 15-30 min; Duration: 60-120 min
    - Fentanyl (analgesia)
        - Loading/bolus dose: 0.35-1.5 mcg/kg IV
        - Infusion (maintenance): 25 mcg/hr, titrate by 25 mcg/hr q15 min
        - Onset: 1 min; Duration: 30 min-1 hr
- If shivering continues despite aggressive sedation, consider a neuromuscular blockade.
    - Cisatracurium
        - Loading dose: 0.15-0.20 mg/kg IV
        - Infusion: 0.5-10.2 mcg/kg/min
        - Onset: 2-3 min; Peak: 3-5 min; Duration: 20-35 min
    - Vecuronium:
        - Loading dose: 0.08-0.1 mg/kg IV

- Infusion (maintenance): 0.8-1.2 mcg/kg/min 40 min later
- Onset: 3-5 min; Duration: 25-40 min

Maintenance phase
- Ice-cold fluids **PLUS** ice packs or cooling blankets can be effective.
- Endovascular catheters with closed feedback technology if available.
- Monitor for complications:
  - Arrhythmias
    - Symptomatic bradycardia (HR<50)
      - Atropine: 0.5 mg IV push every 3-5 min, max dose: 3 mg
    - Stable supraventricular tachycardia
      - Adenosine: 6 mg rapid IV push; can repeat with 12 mg-dose twice if needed.
    - Stable-wide complex tachycardia
      - Procainamide: 20-50 mg/min IV until:
        - ◆ Arrhythmia terminated, hypotension, QRS increases by >50%
        - ◆ Infusion: 1-4 mg/min IV infusion up to max dose 17 mg/kg (*Truncated dosing regimen; refer to other chapters for more succinct dosing.*)
        - ◆ Avoid in prolonged QT_c or CHF.
      - Amiodarone: 150 mg IV over 10 min; repeat if VT recurs.
        - ◆ Maintenance: 1 mg/min for first 6 hrs, (**THEN** decrease infusion to 0.5 mg/min x 18 hrs) up to a max dose of 2.2 g per 24 hrs.
  - "Cold diuresis" and electrolyte disturbance
    - Maintain euvolemia.
    - Check electrolytes q3-4 hrs and replete to high-normal levels.
  - Coagulopathy and platelet dysfunction
    - Generally does not require treatment.
    - Antiplatelet/thrombolytic therapy should still be given as appropriate.
  - Hyperglycemia
    - Can occur even in non-diabetics: goal 144-180 mg/dL.
- Hypotension and post-arrest myocardial stunning
  - Optimize preload with IV fluids.
  - Vasopressors
    - Epinephrine: 0.05-0.5 mcg/kg/min
    - Norepinephrine: 0.05-0.5 mcg/kg/min
  - Inotropes
    - Dobutamine: 5-10 mcg/kg/min, up to max dose of 40 mcg/min
    - Milrinone: Load 50 mcg/kg over 10 min, **THEN** infuse at 0.375-0.75 mcg/kg/min.

PEARLS
→ **MUST** prevent hyperthermia; (morbidity increases with every degree over 37°C).
→ Seizures are common (5-20%); strongly consider EEG monitoring, treat aggressively.
→ Cardiac catheterization is safe during TTM.
→ Avoid hypotension; even a single episode can worsen outcome.

Appendix

Ramsay Sedation Score	
I:	Nervous, agitated, and/or restless
II:	Cooperative, orientated, quiet
III:	Only obeying orders
IV:	Sleeping, brisk response to stimuli
V:	Sleeping, slow response to stimuli
VI:	No response

Riker Sedation-Agitation Score	
7:	Dangerous agitation: pulling at ETT/lines, thrashing
6:	Very agitated: needs restraint, verbal reminders
5:	Agitated: anxious, calms to verbal instructions
4:	Calm/Cooperative: easily aroused, follows commands
3:	Sedated: awake to verbal, simple commands; drifts off
2:	Very sedated: awake to physical stimuli only, no commands
1:	Unarousable: minimal or no response to noxious stimuli

Richmond Agitation-Sedation Scale (RASS)	
+4	Combative: overtly combative, violent, immediate danger to staff
+3	Very agitated: pulls or removes tubes or catheters, aggressive
+2	Agitated: frequent non-purposeful movement, fights ventilator
+1	Restless: anxious, but movements not aggressive or vigorous
0	Alert and calm
-1	Drowsy: not fully alert, but has sustained awakening (eye-opening/eye contact) to *voice* (**>10 sec**)
-2	Light sedation: briefly awakens with eye contact to *voice* (**<10 sec**)
-3	Moderate sedation: movement or eye opening to *voice* (**but no eye contact**)
-4	Deep sedation: no response to voice, but movement or eye opening to *physical* stimulation
-5	Unarousable: no response to *voice or physical* stimulation

References
Chapters listed in alphabetical order

Abdominal Aortic Aneurysm Rupture

Clinical policy: critical issues for the initial evaluation and management of patients presenting with a chief complaint of nontraumatic acute abdominal pain. *Ann Emerg Med* 2000;36: 406-15.

Dick F, Erdoes G, Opfermann P, Eberle B, Schmidli J, Von allmen RS. Delayed volume resuscitation during initial management of ruptured abdominal aortic aneurysm. *J Vasc Surg.* 2013;57(4):943-50.

Powell JT, Thompson SG, Thompson MM, et al. The Immediate Management of the Patient with Rupture: Open Versus Endovascular repair (IMPROVE) aneurysm trial – ISRCTN 48334791 IMPROVE trialists. *Acta Chir Belg* 2009;109:678-80.

Reed K, Curtis L. Aortic emergencies – Part II: Abdominal aneurysms and aortic trauma. www.ebmedicine.net 2006; 8: 3.

Rinckenbach S, Albertini JN, Thaveau F, et al. Prehospital treatment of infrarenal ruptured abdominal aortic aneurysms: a multicentric analysis. *Ann Vasc Surg* 2010;24:308-14.

Acetaminophen Overdose

Bernal W, Donaldson N, Duncan W, Wendon J. Blood lactate as an early predictor of outcome in paracetamol-induced acute liver failure: a cohort study. *The Lancet.* 2002; 359:558-563.

Bond GR, Ho M, Woodward RW. Trends in hepatic injury associated with unintentional overdose of paracetamol (Acetaminophen) in products with and without opioid: an analysis using the National Poison Data System of the American Association of Poison Control Centers, 2000-7. *Drug Saf* 2012;35:149-57.

Hendrickson RG, Bizovi KE. Acetaminophen.inHoffman RS, Nelson LS, GoldfrankLR, Howland MA, Lewin NA, Flomenbaum NE eds. *Goldfrank'sToxicologic Emergencies 9th ed.* McGraw-Hill 2011: 544.

Howland MA. N-acetylcysteine. Hoffman RS, Nelson LS, GoldfrankLR, Howland MA, Lewin NA, Flomenbaum NE eds. *Goldfrank'sToxicologic Emergencies 9th ed.* McGraw-Hill 2011: 500.

Schmidt LA, Dalhoff K. Serum phosphate is an early predictor of outcome in severe acetaminophen-induced hepatotoxicity. *Hepatology.* 2002; 36(3):659-665.

Acute Coronary Syndrome

Anderson JL, Adams CD, Antman EM, et al. ACC/AHA 2007 guidelines for the management of patients with unstable angina/non-ST-Elevation myocardial infarction: a report of the American College of Cardiology/American Heart Association Task Force on Practice Guidelines (Writing Committee to Revise the 2002 Guidelines for the Management of Patients With Unstable Angina/Non-ST-Elevation Myocardial Infarction) developed in collaboration with the American College of Emergency Physicians, the Society for Cardiovascular Angiography and Interventions, and the Society of Thoracic Surgeons endorsed by the American Association of Cardiovascular and Pulmonary Rehabilitation and the Society for Academic Emergency Medicine. *J Am Coll Cardiol* 2007;50: e1-e157.

Hamm CW, Bassand JP, Agewall S, et al. ESC Guidelines for the management of acute coronary syndromes in patients presenting without persistent ST-segment elevation: The Task Force for the management of acute coronary syndromes (ACS) in patients presenting without persistent ST-segment elevation of the European Society of Cardiology (ESC). *Eur Heart J* 2011;32:2999-3054.

O'Gara PT, Kushner FG, Ascheim DD, et al. 2013 ACCF/AHA Guideline for the Management of ST-Elevation Myocardial Infarction: A Report of the American College of Cardiology Foundation/American Heart Association Task Force on Practice Guidelines. *J Am Coll Cardiol.* 2013;61(4):e78-e140.

Trost JC, Lange RA. Treatment of acute coronary syndrome: Part 1: Non-ST-segment acute coronary syndrome. *Crit Care Med* 2011;39:2346-53.

Trost JC, Lange RA. Treatment of acute coronary syndrome: part 2: ST-segment elevation myocardial infarction. *Crit Care Med* 2012;40:1939-45.

Acute Ischemic Stroke

Adams HP, Jr., del Zoppo G, Alberts MJ, et al. Guidelines for the early management of adults with ischemic stroke: a guideline from the American Heart Association/American Stroke Association Stroke Council, Clinical Cardiology Council, Cardiovascular Radiology and Intervention Council, and the Atherosclerotic Peripheral Vascular Disease and Quality of Care Outcomes in Research Interdisciplinary Working Groups: the American Academy of Neurology affirms the value of this guideline as an educational tool for neurologists. *Stroke* 2007;38(5):1655-711.

Clinical Policy: Use of intravenous tPA for the management of acute ischemic stroke in the emergency department. *Ann Emerg Med* 2013;61(2):225-43.

Hacke W, Kaste M, Bluhmki E, et al. Thrombolysis with alteplase 3 to 4.5 hours after acute ischemic stroke. *N Engl J Med* 2008;359(13):1317-29.

Jauch EC, Cucchiara B, Adeoye O, et al. Part 11: adult stroke: 2010 American Heart Association Guidelines for Cardiopulmonary Resuscitation and Emergency Cardiovascular Care. *Circulation* 2010;122(18 Suppl 3):S818-28.

Tissue plasminogen activator for acute ischemic stroke. The National Institute of Neurological Disorders and Stroke rt-PA Stroke Study Group. *N Engl J Med* 1995;333(24):1581-7.

Alcohol Withdrawal Syndrome

Darrouj J, Puri N, Prince E, Lomonaco A, Spevetz A, Gerber DR. Dexmedetomidine infusion as adjunctive therapy to benzodiazepines for acute alcohol withdrawal. *Ann Pharmacother* 2008;42:1703-5.

Hendey GW, Dery RA, Barnes RL, Snowden B, Mentler P. A prospective, randomized, trial of phenobarbital versus benzodiazepines for acute alcohol withdrawal. *Am J Emerg Med* 2011;29:382-5.

Hendey GW, Dery RA, Barnes RL, Snowden B, Mentler P. A prospective, randomized, trial of phenobarbital versus benzodiazepines for acute alcohol withdrawal. *Am J Emerg Med* 2011;29:382-5.

Saitz R, Mayo-Smith MF, Roberts MS, Redmond HA, Bernard DR, Calkins DR. Individualized treatment for alcohol withdrawal. A randomized double-blind controlled trial. *JAMA* 1994;272:519-23.

Anaphylaxis

Dhami S, Panesar SS, Roberts G, et al. Management of anaphylaxis: a systematic review. *Allergy* 2014; 69: 168-175.

Limsuwan T, Demoly P. Acute symptoms of drug hypersensitivity (urticaria, angioedema, anaphylaxis, anaphylactic shock). *Med Clin North Am* 2010;94:691-710, x.

Schummer C, Wirsing M, Schummer W. The pivotal role of vasopressin in refractory anaphylactic shock. *Anesth Analg* 2008;107:620-4.

Simons FE. 2012 update: World allergy organization guidelines for the assessment and management of anaphylaxis. Current opinion in allergy and clinical immunology. 2012;12(4):389-99.

Simons FE. World allergy organization anaphylaxis guidelines: 2013 update of the evidence base. *Int Arch Allergy Immunol.* 2013;162(3):193-204.

Aneurysmal Subarachnoid Hemorrhage

Connolly ES, Jr., Rabinstein AA, Carhuapoma JR, et al. Guidelines for the management of aneurysmal subarachnoid hemorrhage: a guideline for healthcare professionals from the American Heart Association/american Stroke Association. *Stroke* 2012;43(6):1711-37.

Diringer MN. Management of aneurysmal subarachnoid hemorrhage. *Crit Care Med* 2009;37(2):432-440.

Diringer MN, Bleck TP, Claude Hemphill J, 3rd, et al. Critical care management of patients following aneurysmal subarachnoid hemorrhage: recommendations from the Neurocritical Care Society's Multidisciplinary Consensus Conference. *Neurocrit Care* 2011;15(2):211-40.

Edlow JA, Malek AM, Ogilvy CS. Aneurysmal subarachnoid hemorrhage: update for emergency physicians. *J Emerg Med* 2008;34(3):237-51.

Green DM, Burns JD, Defusco CM. Management of aneurysmal subarachnoid hemorrhage. *J Intensive Care Med* 2012;28(6):341-54.

Anticholinergic Toxicity

Anticholinergics and antihistamines. In: Shannon MW, Borron SW, Burns MJ, eds. *Hadded and Winchester's Clinical Management of Poisoning and Drug Overdose.* 4th ed. Philadelphia; Saunders Elsevier; 2007:721-734.

Beaver KM, Gavin TJ. Treatment of acute anticholinergic poisoning with physostigmine. *Am J Emerg Med* 1998;16:505-7.

Burns MJ, Linden CH, Graudins A, Brown RM, Fletcher KE. A comparison of physostigmine and benzodiazepines for the treatment of anticholinergic poisoning. *Ann Emerg Med* 2000;35:374-81.

Kirk KM, Baer AB. Anticholinergics and antihistamines. In: Shannon MW, Borron SW, Burns MJ, eds. *Hadded and Winchester's Clinical Management of Poisoning and Drug Overdose.* 4th ed. Philadelphia; Saunders Elsevier; 2007:721-734.

Anticoagulation

Adams HP Jr, del Zoppo G, Alberts MJ, et al. Guidelines for the early management of adults with ischemic stroke. *Stroke.* May 2007; 38:1655-711.

Jaff MR, McMurty MS, Archer SL, et al. Management of massive and submassive pulmonary embolism, ileofemoral deep vein thrombosis, and chronic thromboembolic pulmonary hypertension: a scientific statement from the American Heart Association. *Circulation.* 2011; 123:1788-830.

Jneid H, Anderson JL, Wright RS, et al. 2012 ACCF/AHA focused update of the guideline for the management of patients with unstable angina/non ST-elevation myocardial infarction. *J Am Coll Cardiol.* 2012; 60:645-81.

Rupprecht HJ, Blank R. Clinical pharmacology of direct and indirect factor Xa inhibitors. *Drugs.* 2010; 70:2153-2170.

The NINDS rt-PA Stroke Study Group. Tissue plasminogen activator for acute ischemic stroke. The National Institute of Neurological Disorders and Stroke rt-PA Stroke Study Group. *N Engl J Med.* 1995; 333:1581-7.

Anticoagulation Reversal

Eerenberg ES, Kamphuisen PW, Sijpkens MK, Meijers JC, Buller HR, Levi M. Reversal of rivaroxaban and dabigatran by prothrombin complex concentrate: a randomized, placebo-controlled, crossover study in healthy subjects. *Circulation.* 2011;124(14):1573-9.

Guyatt GH, Norris SL, Schulman S, et al. Methodology for the development of antithrombotic therapy and prevention of thrombosis guidelines: Antithrombotic Therapy and Prevention of Thrombosis, 9th ed: American College of Chest Physicians Evidence-Based Clinical Practice Guidelines. *Chest.* 2012;141(2 Suppl):53S-70S.

Kumar R, et al J Intensive Care Medicine. March 25 2014 A Review of and Recommendations for the Management of Patients With Life-Threatening Dabigatran-Associated Hemorrhage: A Single-Center University Hospital Experience.

Leissinger CA, Blatt PM, Hoots WK, Ewenstein B. Role of prothrombin complex concentrates in reversing warfarin anticoagulation: a review of the literature. *Am J Hematol* 2008;83:137-43.

Yorkgitis BK, Ruggia-check C, Dujon JE. Antiplatelet and anticoagulation medications and the surgical patient. *Am J Surg.* 2014;207(1):95-101.

Aortic Dissection

Hagan PG, Nienaber CA, Isselbacher EM, et al. The international registry of acute aortic dissection (IRAD): new insights into an old disease. *JAMA* 2000;283:897-903.

Hiratzka LF, Bakris GL, Beckman JA, et al. 2010 ACCF/AHA/AATS/ACR/ASA/SCA/ SCAI/SIR/ STS/SVM guidelines for the diagnosis and management of patients with Thoracic Aortic Disease: a report of the American College of Cardiology Foundation/ American Heart Association Task Force on Practice Guidelines, American Association for Thoracic Surgery, American College of Radiology, American Stroke Association, Society of Cardiovascular Anesthesiologists, Society for Cardiovascular Angiography and Interventions, Society of Interventional Radiology, Society of Thoracic Surgeons, and Society for Vascular Medicine. *Circulation* 2010;121:e266-369.

Marik PE, Rivera R. Hypertensive emergencies: an update. *Curr Opin Crit Care* 2011;17:569-80.

Wittels K. Aortic emergencies. *Emerg Med Clin North Am* 2011;29:789-800, vii.

Atrial Fibrillation with RVR

Demircan C, Cikriklar HI, Engindeniz Z, et al. Comparison of the effectiveness of intravenous diltiazem and metoprolol in the management of rapid ventricular rate in atrial fibrillation. *Emerg Med J* 2005;22:411-4.

Fuster V, Ryden LE, Cannom DS, et al. ACC/AHA/ESC 2006 guidelines for the management of patients with atrial fibrillation — executive summary: a report of the American College of Cardiology/American Heart Association Task Force on Practice Guidelines and the European Society of Cardiology Committee for Practice Guidelines (Writing Committee to Revise the 2001 Guidelines for the Management of Patients With Atrial Fibrillation). *J Am Coll Cardiol* 2006;48:854-906.

Neumar RW, Otto CW, Link MS, et al. Part 8: adult advanced cardiovascular life support: 2010 American Heart Association Guidelines for Cardiopulmonary Resuscitation and Emergency Cardiovascular Care. *Circulation* 2010;122:S729-67.

Schreck DM, Rivera AR, Tricarico VJ. Emergency management of atrial fibrillation and flutter: intravenous diltiazem versus intravenous digoxin. *Ann Emerg Med* 1997;29: 135-40.

Siu CW, Lau CP, Lee WL, Lam KF, Tse HF. Intravenous diltiazem is superior to intravenous amiodarone or digoxin for achieving ventricular rate control in patients with acute uncomplicated atrial fibrillation. *Crit Care Med* 2009;37:2174-9; quiz 2180.

Beta-blocker Overdose

Bailey B. Glucagon in beta-blocker and calcium channel blocker overdoses: a systematic review. *J Toxicol Clin Toxicol.* 2003;41(5):595-602.

Engebretsen KM, Kaczmarek KM, Morgan J, Holger JS. High-dose insulin therapy in beta-blocker and calcium channel-blocker poisoning. *Clin Toxicol* (Phila). 2011;49(4):277-83.

Masson R, Colas V, Parienti JJ, et al. A comparison of survival with and without extracorporeal life support treatment for severe poisoning due to drug intoxication. *Resuscitation.* 2012;83(11):1413-7.

Shepherd G. Treatment of poisoning caused by beta-adrenergic and calcium-channel blockers. *Am J Health Syst Pharm.* 2006;63(19):1828-35.

Tabone D, Ferguson C. BET2: Intralipid/lipid emulsion in beta-blocker overdose. *Emerg Med J.* Nov 2011;28(11):991-3.

Calcium-channel Blocker Overdose

DeRoos FJ. Chapter 60. Calcium Channel Blockers. In: Goldfrank LR, Nelson LS, Hoffman RS, Lewin NA, Howland MA, Flomenbaum NE, eds. *Goldfrank's Toxicologic Emergencies.* 9th ed. New York: McGraw-Hill; 2011.

Durward A, Guerguerian AM, Lefebvre M, Shemie SD. Massive diltiazem overdose treated with extracorporeal membrane oxygenation. *Pediatr Crit Care Med.* Jul 2003;4(3):372-6.

Engebretsen KM, Kaczmarek KM, Morgan J, Holger JS. High-dose insulin therapy in beta-blocker and calcium channel-blocker poisoning. *Clin Toxicol* (Phila) 2011;49:277-83.

Roberts DJ. Chapter 150. Cardiovascular Drugs. In: Marx J, Hockberger R, Walls R, eds. *Rosen's Emergency Medicine: Concepts and Clinical Practice.* 7th ed. Philadelphia: Mosby-Elsevier; 2009

Shepherd G. Treatment of poisoning caused by beta-adrenergic and calcium-channel blockers. *Am J Health Syst Pharm* 2006;63:1828-35.

Cerebral Edema

Broderick J, Connolly S, Feldmann, et al. Guidelines for the Management of Spontaneous Intracerebral Hemorrhage in Adults: 2007 Update: A Guideline From the American Heart Association/American Stroke Association Stroke Council, High Blood Pressure Research Council, and the Quality of Care and Outcomes in Research Interdisciplinary Working Group: The American Academy of Neurology affirms the value of this guideline as an educational tool for neurologists. *Stroke.* 2007;38:2001-2023.

Francony G, Fauvage B, Falcon D, et al. Equimolar doses of mannitol and hypertonic saline in the treatment of increased intracranial pressure. *Crit Care Med* 2008;36:795- 800.

Kamel H, Navi BB, Nakagawa K, Hemphill JC, 3rd, Ko NU. Hypertonic saline versus mannitol for the treatment of elevated intracranial pressure: a meta-analysis of randomized clinical trials. *Crit Care Med* 2011;39:554-9.

Morgenstern LB, Hemphill JC, 3rd, Anderson C, et al. Guidelines for the management of spontaneous intracerebral hemorrhage: a guideline for healthcare professionals from the American Heart Association/American Stroke Association. *Stroke* 2010;41:2108-29.

Szaflarski JP, Sangha KS, Lindsell CJ, Shutter LA. Prospective, randomized, single-blinded comparative trial of intravenous levetiracetam versus phenytoin for seizure prophylaxis. *Neurocrit Care* 2010;12:165-72

Cholinergic Crisis

Abedin MJ, Sayeed AA, Basher A, et al. Open-label randomized clinical trial of atropine bolus injection versus incremental boluses plus infusion for organophosphate poisoning in Bangladesh. *J Med Toxicol* 2012; 8:108.

Agency for Toxic Substances and Disease Registry (ATSDR), "Medical Management Guidelines for Nerve Agents: Tabun (GA); Sarin (GB); Soman (GD); and VX," August, 2008. Available at www.atsdr.cdc.gov/mhmi/mmg166.pdf Accessed on 2/15/2012.

Blain PG. Organophosphorous poisoning (acute). Clinical evidence 2011; 2011.

Indira M, Andrews MA, Rakesh TP. Incidence, predictors, and outcome of intermediate syndrome in cholinergic insecticide poisoning: a prospective observational cohort study. *Clin Toxicol.* 2013; 51:838.

Pawar KS, Bhoite RR, Pillay CP, et al. Continuous pralidoxime infusion versus repeated bolus injection to treat organophosphorus pesticide poisoning: a randomised controlled trial. *Lancet.* Dec 16 2006; 368 (9553): 2136-2141.

Coagulopathy Reversal

Hunt BJ. Bleeding and coagulopathies in critical care. N Engl J Med. 2014;370(9):847-59.

Fauci AS. Harrison's Principles of Internal Medicine. New York: McGraw-Hill Medical, c2008.; 2012.

Marx JA, Hockberger RS, Walls RM. Rosen's Emergency Medicine – Concepts and Clinical Practice, Edition 7. Elsevier Health Sciences; 2009.

Linkins LA, Dans AL, Moores LK, et al. Treatment and prevention of heparin-induced thrombocytopenia: Antithrombotic Therapy and Prevention of Thrombosis, 9th ed: American College of Chest Physicians Evidence-Based Clinical Practice Guidelines. *Chest.* 2012;141(2 Suppl):e495S-530S.

Congestive Heart Failure

Bart BA, Boyle A, Bank AJ, et al. Ultrafiltration versus usual care for hospitalized patients with heart failure: the Relief for Acutely Fluid-Overloaded Patients With Decompensated Congestive Heart Failure (RAPID-CHF) trial. *J Am Coll Cardiol* 2005;46:2043-6.

Felker GM, Lee KL, Bull DA, et al. Diuretic strategies in patients with acute decompensated heart failure. *N Engl J Med* 2011;364:797-805.

Hunt SA, Abraham WT, Chin MH, et al. 2009 focused update incorporated into the ACC/ AHA 2005 Guidelines for the Diagnosis and Management of Heart Failure in Adults: a report of the American College of Cardiology Foundation/American Heart Association Task Force on Practice Guidelines: developed in collaboration with the International Society for Heart and Lung Transplantation. *Circulation* 2009;119:e391-479.

Marik PE, Flemmer M. Narrative review: the management of acute decompensated heart failure. *J Intensive Care Med.* 2012;27(6):343-53.

Peacock WF, Hollander JE, Diercks DB, Lopatin M, Fonarow G, Emerman CL. Morphine and outcomes in acute decompensated heart failure: an ADHERE analysis. *Emerg Med J.* 2008;25(4):205-9.

Cyanide Toxicity

Bebarta VS, Tanen DA, Lairet J, Dixon PS, Valtier S, Bush A. Hydroxocobalamin and sodium thiosulfate versus sodium nitrite and sodium thiosulfate in the treatment of acute cyanide toxicity in a swine (Sus scrofa) model. *Ann Emerg Med* 2010;55:345-51.

Borron SW, Baud FJ, Megarbane B, Bismuth C. Hydroxocobalamin for severe acute cyanide poisoning by ingestion or inhalation. *Am J Emerg Med* 2007;25:551-8.

Hall AH, Dart R, Bogdan G. Sodium thiosulfate or hydroxocobalamin for the empiric treatment of cyanide poisoning? *Ann Emerg Med* 2007;49:806-13.

O'Brien DJ, Walsh DW, Terriff CM, Hall AH. Empiric management of cyanide toxicity associated with smoke inhalation. *Prehosp Disaster Med* 2011;26:374-82.

Streitz MJ, Bebarta VS, Borys DJ, Morgan DL. Patterns of Cyanide Antidote Use Since Regulatory Approval of Hydroxocobalamin in the United States. *Am J Ther* 2013 May 17.

Diabetic Ketoacidosis

Global IDF:ISPAD guideline for diabetes in childhood and adolescence. Available at: www.idf.org/sites/default/files/Diabetes-in-Childhood-and-Adolescence-Guidelines. Accessed January 2, 2014.

Goyal N, Miller JB, Sankey SS, Mossallam U. Utility of initial bolus insulin in the treatment of diabetic ketoacidosis. *J Emerg Med.* 2010;38:422-427.

Kitabchi AE, Umpierrez GE, Murphy MB, Kreisberg RA. Hyperglycemic crises in adult patients with diabetes: a consensus statement from the American Diabetes Association. *Diabetes Care.* 2006;29:2739-2748.

Nygenwe E. and Kitabchi, A. Evidence-based management of hyperglycemic emergencies in diabetes mellitus. *Diab clin prac.* 2011;94:340-351.

Van Ness-Otunnu, R. and Hack. J. Hyperglycemic Crisis. *J Emerg Med.* 2013;45(5):797-805.

Digoxin Toxicity

Antman EM, Wenger TL, Butler VP, Jr., Haber E, Smith TW. Treatment of 150 cases of life-threatening digitalis intoxication with digoxin-specific Fab antibody fragments. Final report of a multicenter study. *Circulation* 1990;81:1744-52.

Bateman DN. Digoxin-specific antibody fragments: how much and when? *Toxicol Rev* 2004; 23:135-43.

Bauman JL, DiDomenico RJ, Galanter WL. Mechanisms, manifestations, and management of digoxin toxicity the modern era. *American Journal of Cardiovascular Drugs* 2006;6:77-86.

European Heart Rhythm Association, Heart Rhythm Society, D.P. Zipes, A.J. Camm, M. Borggrefe, A.E. Buxton, B. Chaitman, M. Fromer, G. Gregoratos, G. Klein, A.J. Moss, R.J. Myerburg, S.G. Priori, M.A. Quinones, D.M. Roden et al. ACC/AHA/ESC 2006 guidelines for management of patients with ventricular arrhythmias and the prevention of sudden cardiac death: a report of the American College of Cardiology/American Heart Association Task Force and the European Society of Cardiology Committee for Practice Guidelines (Writing Committee to Develop Guidelines for Management of Patients With Ventricular Arrhythmias and the Prevention of Sudden Cardiac Death) *J Am Coll Cardiol* 2006;48:e247–e346.

Eclampsia

American College of Obstetricians and Gynecologists. Hypertension in Pregnancy, developed by the Task Force on Hypertension in Pregnancy, Nov 2013

American College of Obstetricians and Gynecologists. Emergent therapy for acute-onset, severe hypertension with preeclampsia or eclampsia. Committee Opinion No. 514. *Obstet Gynecol.* Dec 2011;118:1465-8.

Tompkins MJ, Thiagarajah S. HELLP (hemolysis, elevated liver enzymes, and low platelet count) syndrome: the benefit of corticosteroids. *Am J Obstet Gynecol.* Aug 1999;181(2):304-9.

Hydrofluoric Acid Toxicity

Baltazar RF, Mower MM, Reider R, Funk M, Salomon J. Acute fluoride poisoning leading to fatal hyperkalemia. *Chest* 1980;78:660-3.

Bartlett D. Dermal exposure to hydrofluoric acid causing significant systemic toxicity. *J Emerg Nurs* 2004;30:371-3.

Dalamaga M, Karmaniolas K, Nikolaidou A, Papadavid E. Hypocalcemia, hypomagnesemia, and hypokalemia following hydrofluoric acid chemical injury. *J Burn Care Res* 2008;29:541-3.

Hojer J, Personne M, Hulten P, Ludwigs U. Topical treatments for hydrofluoric acid burns: a blind controlled experimental study. *J Toxicol Clin Toxicol* 2002;40:861-6.

Wedler V, Guggenheim M, Moron M, Kunzj W, Meyer VE. Extensive hydrofluoric acid injuries: a serious problem. *J Trauma* 2005;58:852-7.

Hypernatremia

Arora SK. Hypernatremic Disorders in the Intensive Care Unit. J Intensive Care Med 2011.

Lee JW. Fluid and electrolyte disturbances in critically ill patients. *Electrolyte Blood Press* 2010;8:72-81.

Kraft MD, Btaiche IF, Sacks GS, Kudsk KA. Treatment of electrolyte disorders in adult patients in the intensive care unit. *Am J Health Syst Pharm* 2005;62:1663-82.

Hypertensive Emergency

Flanigan JS, Vitberg D. Hypertensive emergency and severe hypertension: what to treat, who to treat, and how to treat. *Med Clin North Am* 2006;90:439-51.

Marik PE, Rivera R. Hypertensive emergencies: an update. *Curr Opin Crit Care* 2011;17:569-80.

Hyponatremia

Adrogue HJ, Madias NE. Hyponatremia. *N Engl J Med.* 2000 May 25;342(21):1581-9.

Moritz, ML, Ayus JC. 100 cc 3% sodium chloride bolus: a novel treatment for hyponatremic encephalopathy. *Metab Brain Dis.* 2010 Mar;25(1):91-6.

Pfennig CL, Slovis CM. Sodium Disorders in the emergency department: a review of hyponatremia and hypernatremia. *Emerg Med Pract.* 2012 Oct;14(10):1-26.

Sterns RH, Hix JK, Silver S. Treating profound hyponatremia: a strategy for controlled correction. *Am J Kidney Dis.* 2010 Oct;56(4):774-9.

Verbalis JG, Goldsmith SR, Greenberg A, et al. Diagnosis, evaluation, and treatment of hyponatremia: expert panel recommendations. *Am J Med.* 2013 Oct;126(10 Suppl 1):S1-42.

Mesenteric Ischemia

Bergqvist D, Svensson PJ. Treatment of mesenteric vein thrombosis. *Semin Vasc Surg.* 2010;23(1):65-8.

Berland T, Oldenburg WA. Acute mesenteric ischemia. *Curr Gastroenterol Rep* 2008;10:341-6.

Oldenburg WA, Lau LL, Rodenberg TJ, Edmonds HJ, Burger CD. Acute mesenteric ischemia: a clinical review. *Arch Intern Med.* 2004;164(10):1054-62.

Theodoropoulou A, Koutroubakis IE. Ischemic colitis: clinical practice in diagnosis and treatment. *World J Gastroenterol.* 2008;14(48):7302-8.

Washington C, Carmichael JC. Management of ischemic colitis. *Clin Colon Rectal Surg.* 2012;25(4):228-35.

Neuroleptic Malignant Syndrome

Bhanushali MJ, Tuite PJ. The evaluation and management of patients with neuroleptic malignant syndrome. *Neurol Clin* 2004;22:389-411.

Carbone JR. The neuroleptic malignant and serotonin syndromes. *Emerg Med Clin North Am* 2000;18:317-25, x.Neuroleptic Malignant Syndrome Information Service. www.nmsis.org, last accessed May 20, 2012

Perry PJ, Wilborn CA. Serotonin syndrome vs neuroleptic malignant syndrome: a contrast of causes, diagnoses, and management. *Ann Clin Psychiatry.* 2012;24(2):155-62.

Strawn JR, Keck PE, Jr., Caroff SN. Neuroleptic malignant syndrome. *Am J Psychiatry* 2007;164:870-6.

Susman VL. Clinical management of neuroleptic malignant syndrome. *Psychiatr Q* 2001;72: 325-36.

Opioid Overdose

Nelson LS. Chapter 38. Opioids. In: Goldfrank LR, Nelson LS, Hoffman RS, Lewin NA, Howland MA, Flomenbaum NE, eds. *Goldfrank's Toxicologic Emergencies.* 9thed. New York: McGraw-Hill; 2011.

Oral Hypoglycemic Overdose

Bosse, GM. "Antidiabetics and Hypoglycemics." In: Goldfrank LR, Nelson LS, Hoffman RS, Lewin NA, Howland MA, Flomenbaum NE, eds. *Goldfrank's Toxicologic Emergencies.* 9th ed. New York: McGraw-Hill; 714-727.

Diamant M, Morsink LM. SGLT2 Inhibitors for diabetes: turning symptoms into therapy. *Lancet.* 2013: 382: 917-8.

Fasano CJ, O'Malley G, Dominici P, Aguilera E, Latta DR. Comparison of octreotide and standard therapy versus standard therapy alone for the treatment of sulfonylurea- induced hypoglycemia. *Ann Emerg Med* 2008;51:400-6.

Lheureux PE, Zahir S, Penaloza A, Gris M. Bench-to-bedside review: Antidotal treatment of sulfonylurea-induced hypoglycaemia with octreotide. *Crit Care* 2005;9:543-9.

Seidowsky A, Nseir S, Houdret N, Fourrier F. Metformin-associated lactic acidosis: a prognostic and therapeutic study. *Crit Care.* 2009;37:2191-6.

Paralytics

Di Filippo A, Gonnelli C. Rapid-sequence intubation: a review of recent evidences. *Rev Recent Clin Trials* 2009;4:175-8.

Greenberg SB, Vender J. The use of neuromuscular blocking agents in the ICU: where are we now? *Crit Care Med.* 2013;41(5):1332-44.

Piriyapatsom A, Bittner EA, Hines J, Schmidt UH. Sedation and paralysis. *Respir Care.* 2013;58(6):1024-37.

Srivastava A, Hunter JM. Reversal of neuromuscular block. *Br J Anaesth* 2009;103:115-29.

Warr J, Thiboutot Z, Rose L, Mehta S, Burry LD. Current therapeutic uses, pharmacology, and clinical considerations of neuromuscular blocking agents for critically ill adults. *Ann Pharmacother* 2011;45:1116-26.

Pediatric Cardiogenic Shock

Brierley J, Carcillo JA, Choong K, et al. Clinical practice parameters for hemodynamic support of pediatric and neonatal septic shock: 2007 update from the American College of Critical Care Medicine. *Crit Care Med* 2009;37:666-88.

Carcillo JA, Han K, Lin JC, Orr RA. Goal-directed management of pediatric shock in the emergency department. *Clin Ped Emerg Med.* 2007:8(3);165-75.

Fisher JD, Nelson DG, Beyersdorf H, Satkowiak LJ. Clinical spectrum of shock in the pediatric emergency department. *Pediatr Emerg Care* 2010;26:622-5.

Kleinman ME, Chameides L, Schexnayder S, et al. Pediatric Advanced Life Support: 2010 American Heart Association Guidelines for Cardiopulmonary Resuscitation and Emergency Cardiovascular Care. *Pediatrics* 2010; 1361 -1389.

Thangaratinam S, Brown K, Zamora J, et al. Pulse oximetry screening for critical congenital heart defects in asymptomatic newborn babies: a systematic review and meta-analysis. *Lancet* 2012: 379(9835):2459-64.

Xiao N, Tandon A, et al. Cardiogenic Shock as the initial presentation of neonatal systemic hypertension. Journal of Neonatal-Peinatal Medicine. 2013; 6:267-272.

Pediatric Sedation

Baxter AL, Mallory MD, Spandorfer PR, et al. Etomidate versus pentobarbital for computed tomography sedations: report from the Pediatric Sedation Research Consortium. *Pediatr Emerg Care.* 2007;23(10):690-5.

Cote CJ, Wilson S. Guidelines for monitoring and management of pediatric patients during and after sedation for diagnostic and therapeutic procedures: an update. *Pediatrics* 2006;118:2587-602.

Cravero JP, Havidich JE. Pediatric sedation — evolution and revolution. *Paediatr Anaesth* 2011;21:800-9.

Madati, J. Ketamine: Pediatric Procedural Sedation in the Emergency Department. *Pediatric Emergency Medicine Practice.* Jan 2011; 8(1):1-20.

Wolfe TR, Braude DA. Intranasal medication delivery for children: a brief review and update. *Pediatrics* 2010;126:532-7.

Pediatric Septic Shock

Brierley J, Peters M. Distinct Hemodynamic Patterns of Septic Shock at Presentation to Pediatric Intensive Care. *Pediatrics*. October 2008; 122: 752-759.

Brierley J, Carcillo JA, Choong K, et al. Clinical practice parameters for hemodynamic support of pediatric and neonatal septic shock: 2007 update from the American College of Critical Care Medicine. *Crit Care Med* 2009;37:666-88.

Dellinger RP, Levy MM, Rhodes A, et al. Surviving Sepsis Campaign: International Guidelines for Management of Severe Sepsis and Sepic Shock: 2012. *Crit Care Med*. 2013 Feb; 41(2):580-637.

Hauser, Gabriel MD, MBA. Early Goal-Directed Therapy for Pediatric Septic Shock in the Emergency Department. Israeli *J Emerg Med*. June 2007 Vol 7, No 2. 5-17.

Parker MM, Hazelzet JA, Carcillo JA. Pediatric Considerations. *Crit Care Med*. 2004; 32: 591-594.

Pit Viper Envenomation

Adukauskiene D, Varanauskiene E, Adukauskaite A. Venomous snakebites. *Medicina (Kaunas)*. 2011; 47(80): 461-7.

Camilleri C, Offerman S. Anaphylaxis after Rattlesnake bite. *Ann Emerg Med*. 2004;43(6): 784-5.

CroFab® (package insert). West Conshohocken, PA. BTG International, Inc 2010.

Keating GM, Lyseng-Williamson KA.Crotalidae Polyvalent Immune Fab: A Guide to Its Use in North American Crotaline Envenomation. *Clin Drug Investig*. 2012; 32(8):555-60.

Lavonas EJ, *et al.* Unified treatment algorithm for the management of crotaline snakebite in the United States: results of an evidence-informed consensus workshop. *BMC Emerg Med.* 2011; 11:2.

Pulmonary Hypertension (PHTN)

Delcroix M, Naeijie R. Optimising the management of pulmonary arterial hypertension patients: emergency treatments. *Eur Respir Rev* 2010;19(117):204-11

Hoeper MM, Granton J. Intensive care unit management of patients with severe pulmonary hypertension and right heart failure. *Am J Resp Crit Care Med* 2011;184(10):1114-24.

Kollef, Isakow. The Washington Manual of Critical Care. *Lippincott Williams & Wilkins* 2012.

Lahm T, McCaslin C, Wosniak T, et al. Medical and surgical treatment of acute right ventricular failure. *J Am Coll Cardiol* 2010;56:1435-46.

Piazza G, Goldhaber S. The acutely decompensated right ventricle: pathways for diagnostic management. *Chest* 2005;128:1836-1852.

Pulmonary Embolism (PE)

Fesmire FM, Brown MD, et al. Critical issues in the evaluation and management of adult patients presenting to the emergency department with suspected pulmonary embolism. *Ann Emerg Med* 2011;57:628-52 e75.

Jaff MR, McMurtry MS, et al. Management of massive and submassive pulmonary embolism, iliofemoral deep vein thrombosis, and chronic thromboembolic pulmonary hypertension: a scientific statement from the American Heart Association. *Circulation* 2011;123:1788-830.

Kearon C, Akl EA, et al. Antithrombotic therapy for VTE disease: Antithrombotic Therapy and Prevention of Thrombosis, 9th ed: American College of Chest Physicians Evidence-Based Clinical Practice Guidelines. *Chest* 2012;141:e419S-94S.

Meyer G, Vicaut E, et al., for PEITHO Investigators. Fibrinolysis for patients with intermediate risk pulmonary embolism. *N Engl J Med* 2014;370:1402-1411.

Sharifi M, Bay C, et al. Moderate Pulmonary Embolism Treated with Thrombolysis (from the "MOPETT" trial). *Am J Cardiol* 2013;111(2):273-7.

Salicylate Toxicity

O'Malley GF. Emergency department management of the salicylate-poisoned patient. *Emerg Med Clin North Am* 2007;25:333-46; abstract viii.

Proudfoot AT, Krenzelok EP, Vale JA. Position Paper on urine alkalinization. *J Toxicol Clin Toxicol* 2004;42:1-26.

Sedation

Andolfatto G, Abu-laban RB, Zed PJ, et al. Ketamine-propofol combination (ketofol) versus propofol alone for emergency department procedural sedation and analgesia: a randomized double-blind trial. *Ann Emerg Med.* 2012;59(6):504-12.e1-2.

Barr J, Fraser GL, Puntillo K, et al. Clinical Practice Guidelines for the Management of Pain, Agitation, and Delirium in Adult Patients in the Intensive Care Unit. *Critical Care Medicine* 2013; 41: 263-306.

Mason MA, Weant KA, Baker SN. Rapid-Sequence Intubation Medication Therapies A review in Light of Recent Drug Shortages. *Advanced Emergency Nursing Journal* 2013; 35: 16-25.

McPhee LC, Badawi O, Fraser GL, et al. Single-dose etomidate is not associated with increased mortality in ICU patients with sepsis: analysis of a large electronic ICU database. *Critical Care Medicine* 2013;41(3):774-83.

Stollings JL, Diedrich DA, Oyen LJ et al. Rapid-Sequence intubation: A Review of the Process and Considerations When Choosing Medications. *Annals of Pharmacotherapy* 2014; 48: 62-76.

Sepsis

De Backer D, Aldecoa C, Njimi H, Vincent JL. Dopamine versus norepinephrine in the treatment of septic shock: a meta-analysis. *Crit Care Med* 2012;40:725-30.

De Backer D, Biston P, Devriendt J, et al. Comparison of dopamine and norepinephrine in the treatment of shock. *N Engl J Med* 2010;362:779-89.

Delaney AP, Dan A, McCaffrey J, Finfer S. The role of albumin as a resuscitation fluid for patients with sepsis: a systematic review and meta-analysis. *Crit Care Med* 2011;39:386-91.

Dellinger, et al. Surviving Sepsis Campaign: International Guidelines for Management of Severe Sepsis and Septic Shock. *Crit Care Med* 2013;41:580-637.

Finfer S, Chittock DR, Su SY, et al. Intensive versus conventional glucose control in critically ill patients. *N Engl J Med* 2009;360:1283-97.

ProCESS Trial Investigators, Yealy DM, Kellum JA, et al. A randomized trial of protocol-based care for early septic shock. *N Engl J Med* 2014; 370(18):1683-93.

Yunos NM, Bellomo R, Hegarty C, et al. Association between a chloride-liberal vs chloride-restrictive intravenous fluid administration strategy and kidney injury in critically ill adults. *JAMA* 2012l308:1566-72.

Single-dose Pressors

Habib AS. A review of the impact of phenylephrine administration on maternal hemodynamics and maternal and neonatal outcomes in women undergoing cesarean delivery under spinal anesthesia. *Anesth Analg* 2012;114:377-90.

Lee A, Ngan Kee WD, Gin T. A quantitative, systematic review of randomized controlled trials of ephedrine versus phenylephrine for the management of hypotension during spinal anesthesia for cesarean delivery. *Anesth Analg* 2002;94:920-6, table of contents.

Ngan Kee WD, Khaw KS, Lau TK, Ng FF, Chui K, Ng KL. Randomised double-blinded comparison of phenylephrine vs ephedrine for maintaining blood pressure during spinal anaesthesia for non-elective Caesarean section. *Anaesthesia* 2008;63:1319-26.

Prakash S, Pramanik V, Chellani H, Salhan S, Gogia AR. Maternal and neonatal effects of bolus administration of ephedrine and phenylephrine during spinal anaesthesia for caesarean delivery: a randomised study. *Int J Obstet Anesth* 2010;19:24-30.

Weingart, Scott, "Upstairs Care Downstairs" *ACEP Clinical Care and Management*. March 2010. Accessed February 22, 2012

Status Asthmaticus

Kim IK, Saville AL, Sikes KL, Corcoran TE. Heliox-driven albuterol nebulization for asthma exacerbations: an overview. *Respir Care* 2006;51:613-8.

National Asthma Education and Prevention Program: Expert Panel Report III: Guidelines for the diagnosis and management of asthma. Bethesda, MD. National Heart, Lung, and Blood Institute, 2007. (NIH publication no. 08-4051) www.nhlbi.nih.gov/guidelines/ asthma/ asthgdln.htm (Accessed on February 11, 2012).

Rodrigo GJ, Castro-Rodriguez JA. Anticholinergics in the treatment of children and adults with acute asthma: a systematic review with meta-analysis. *Thorax* 2005;60:740-6.

Reuben AD, Harris AR. Heliox for asthma in the emergency department: a review of the literature. *Emerg Med J* 2004;21:131-5.

Shlamovitz GZ, Hawthorne T. Intravenous ketamine in a dissociating dose as a temporizing measure to avoid mechanical ventilation in adult patient with severe asthma exacerbation. *J Emerg Med* 2011;41:492-4.

Status Epilepticus

Brophy GM, Bell R, Claassen J, et al. Guidelines for the evaluation and management of status epilepticus. *NeuroCrit Care.* 2012;17(1):3-23.

Huff JS, Melnick ER, Tomaszewski CA, et al. Clinical policy: critical issues in the evaluation and management of adult patients presenting to the emergency department with seizures. *Ann Emerg Med.* 2014;63(4):437-47.e15.

Meierkord H, Holtkamp M. Non-convulsive status epilepticus in adults: clinical forms and treatment. *Lancet* Neurol. 2007;6(4):329-39.

Meierkord H, Boon P, Engelsen B, et al. EFNS guideline on the management of status epilepticus in adults. *Eur J Neurol.* 2010;17(3):348-55.

Wheless JW, Vazquez BR, Kanner AM, Ramsay RE, Morton L, Pellock JM. Rapid infusion with valproate sodium is well tolerated in patients with epilepsy. *Neurology.* 2004;63(8):1507-8.

Supraventricular Tachycardia

Cornell, Singh. Evidenced based approach to SVT. EM Practice 2008; 10: 1-4.

Delacretaz E. Clinical practice. Supraventricular tachycardia. *N Engl J Med* 2006;354: 1039-51.

Graboys TB, Podrid PJ, Lown B. Efficacy of amiodarone for refractory supraventricular tachyarrhythmias. *Am Heart J* 1983;106:870-6.

Trappe HJ, Brandts B, Weismueller P. Arrhythmias in the intensive care patient. *Curr Opin Crit Care* 2003;9:345-55.

Yealy, Donald M; Delbridge, Theodore. Dysrhythmias. *Rosen's Emergency Medicine: Concepts and Clinical Practice, 7th Edition.* Philadelphia: Mosby Elsevier, 2010: 984-1024.

Targeted Temperature Management

Bernard SA, Gray TW, Buist MD, et al. Treatment of comatose survivors of out-of-hospital cardiac arrest with induced hypothermia. *N Engl J Med* 2002;346:557-63.

Choi HA, Ko SB, Presciutti M, et al. Prevention of shivering during therapeutic temperature modulation: the Columbia anti-shivering protocol. *NeuroCrit Care* 2011;14:389-94.

Jacobshagen C, Pax A, Unsold BW, et al. Effects of large volume, ice-cold intravenous fluid infusion on respiratory function in cardiac arrest survivors. *Resuscitation* 2009;80:1223-8.

Neumar RW, Nolan JP, Adrie C, et al. Post-cardiac arrest syndrome: epidemiology, pathophysiology, treatment, and prognostication. A consensus statement from the International Liaison Committee on Resuscitation (American Heart Association, Australian and New Zealand Council on Resuscitation, European Resuscitation Council, Heart and Stroke Foundation of Canada, InterAmerican Heart Foundation, Resuscitation Council of Asia, and the Resuscitation Council of Southern Africa); the American Heart Association Emergency Cardiovascular Care Committee; the Council on Cardiovascular Surgery and Anesthesia; the Council on Cardiopulmonary, Perioperative, and Critical Care; the Council on Clinical Cardiology; and the Stroke Council. *Int Emerg Nurs.* 2010 Jan;18(1):8-28.

Nielsen N, Wettersley J, Cronberg T, et al. Targeted temperature management at 33C versus 36C after cardiac arrest. *N Engl J Med* 2013;369;2197-2206.

Peberdy MA, Callaway CW, Neumar RW, et al. Part 9: post-cardiac arrest care: 2010 American Heart Association Guidelines for Cardiopulmonary Resuscitation and Emergency Cardiovascular Care. *Circulation* 2010;122:S768-86.

Zeiner A, Holzer M, Sterz F, et al. Hyperthermia after cardiac arrest is associated with an unfavorable neurologic outcome. *Arch Intern Med* 2001;161:2007-12.

Toxic Alcohol Ingestion

Arora A. The 'gap' in the 'plasma osmolar gap'. *BMJ Case Rep.* 2013.

Barceloux DG, Bond GR, Krenzelok EP, Cooper H, Vale JA. American Academy of Clinical Toxicology practice guidelines on the treatment of methanol poisoning. *J Toxicol Clin Toxicol* 2002;40:415-46.

Barceloux DG, Krenzelok EP, Olson K, Watson W. American Academy of Clinical Toxicology Practice Guidelines on the Treatment of Ethylene Glycol Poisoning. Ad Hoc Committee. *J Toxicol Clin Toxicol* 1999;37:537-60.

Brent J, McMartin K, Phillips S, Aaron C, Kulig K. Fomepizole for the treatment of methanol poisoning. *N Engl J Med* 2001;344:424-9.

Weiner SW: Toxic Alcohols, in In: Goldfrank LR, Nelson LS, Hoffman RS, Lewin NA, Howland MA, Flomenbaum NE, eds. *Goldfrank's Toxicologic Emergencies.* 9th ed. New York: McGraw-Hill; Chapter 107.

Traumatic Spinal Cord Injury

Bracken MB. Steroids for acute spinal cord injury. *Cochrane Database Syst Rev* 2012;1: CD001046.

Chen HL, Wang XD. Heparin for venous thromboembolism prophylaxis in patients with acute spinal cord injury: a systematic review and meta-analysis. *Spinal Cord* 2013;51(8):596-602.

Consortium for Spinal Cord Medicine. Early acute management in adults with spinal cord injury: a clinical practice guideline for health-care professionals. *Spinal Cord Med* 2008;May:1-69.

Hadley MN. Blood pressure management after acute spinal cord injury. *Neurosurgery* 2002; 50 (3 Suppl):S58-62.

Hulbert RJ, Hadley MN, Walters BC, Aarabi B, Dhall SS, Gelb DE, Rozzelle CJ, Ryken TC, Theodore N. Pharmacological therapy after acute cervical spinal cord injury. *Neurosurgery* 2013;72:93–105.

Jia X, Kowalski RG, Sciubba DM, Geocadin RG. Critical care of traumatic spinal cord injury. *J Intensive Care Med* 2013;28(1):12-23.

Tricyclic Antidepressant Overdose

Benowitz NL. Antidepressants, Tricyclic. In: Olson KR, ed. *Poisoning & Drug Overdose*. 5th ed. New York: McGraw-Hill; 2007.

Blackman K, Brown SG, Wilkes GJ. Plasma alkalinization for tricyclic antidepressant toxicity: a systematic review. *Emerg Med* (Fremantle) 2001;13:204-10.

Boehnert MT, Lovejoy FH, Jr. Value of the QRS duration versus the serum drug level in predicting seizures and ventricular arrhythmias after an acute overdose of tricyclic antidepressants. *N Engl J Med* 1985;313:474-9.

Body R, Bartram T, Azam F, Mackway-jones K. Guidelines in Emergency Medicine Network (GEMNet): guideline for the management of tricyclic antidepressant overdose. *Emerg Med J*. 2011;28(4):347-68.

Liebelt EL, Francis PD. Cyclic Antidepressants. In: Goldfrank LR, Nelson LS, Hoffman RS, Lewin NA, Howland MA, Flomenbaum NE, eds. *Goldfrank's Toxicologic Emergencies*. 9th ed. New York: McGraw-Hill.

Tumor Lysis Syndrome

McDonnell, AM, Lenz KL, Frei-Lahr, DA, et al. Single-dose rasburicase 6 mg in the management of tumor lysis syndrome in adults. *Pharmacotherapy* 2006: 26:806.

Coiffier, B, Altman, A, Ching-Hon, P, et al. Guidelines for the management of pediatric and adult tumor lysis syndrome: an evidence-based review. *J Onc*. June 2008; 26 (16): 2767-2778.

Parham, W, Mehdirad, A, et al. Revisiting hyperkaelmia. *Tex Heart Inst J* 2006;33:40-7.

Tosi P, Barosi G, Lazzaro C, et al. Consensus conference on the management of tumor lysis syndrome. *Haematologica* 2008;93:1877-1855.

Wilson FP, Berns JS. Tumor lysis syndrome: new challenges and recent advances. *Adv Chronic Kidney Dis* 2014;21:18-26.

Upper GI Bleed

Barkun AN, Bardou M, Kuipers EJ, et al. International consensus recommendations on the management of patients with nonvariceal upper gastrointestinal bleeding. *Ann Intern Med* 2010;152:101-13.

Garcia-Tsao G, Bosch J. Management of varices and variceal hemorrhage in cirrhosis. *N Engl J Med* 2010;362:823-32.

Villanueva C, Colomo A, Bosch A, et al. Transfusion Strategies for Acute Upper Gastrointestinal Bleeding. *N Engl J Med*. 2013; 368(1):11-21.

Ventricular Tachycardia

Neumar RW, Otto CW, Link MS, et al. Part 8: adult advanced cardiovascular life support: 2010 American Heart Association Guidelines for Cardiopulmonary Resuscitation and Emergency Cardiovascular Care. *Circulation* 2010;122:S729-67.

Ward, K, Neumar, R. Adult Resuscitation. *Rosen's Emergency Medicine: Concepts and Clinical Practice, 7th Edition*. Philadelphia: Mosby Elsevier, 2010: 984-1024.

Zipes DP, Camm AJ, Borggrefe M, et al. ACC/AHA/ESC 2006 Guidelines for Management of Patients With Ventricular Arrhythmias and the Prevention of Sudden Cardiac Death: a report of the American College of Cardiology/American Heart Association Task Force and the European Society of Cardiology Committee for Practice Guidelines (writing committee to develop Guidelines for Management of Patients With Ventricular Arrhythmias and the Prevention of Sudden Cardiac Death): developed in collaboration with the European Heart Rhythm Association and the Heart Rhythm Society. *Circulation* 2006;114:e385-484.

Shepherd G. Treatment of poisoning caused by beta-adrenergic and calcium-channel blockers. *Am J Health Syst Pharm* 2006;63:1828-35.

Index